Livestock Update

LIVESTOCK UPDATE

Editors :

UMESH SINGH, RAJIB DEB
SUSHIL KUMAR & ARJAVA SHARMA

Project Directorate on Cattle (ICAR)
Grass Farm Road, Meerut-250 001
Uttar Pradesh (India)

SSPH

SATISH SERIAL PUBLISHING HOUSE

403, Express Tower, Commercial Complex, Azadpur, Delhi-110033 (India)
Phone : 011-27672852, Fax : 91-11-27672046
E-mail :info@satishserial.com, hkjain1975@yahoo.com
Website : www.satishserial.com

Published by :

SATISH SERIAL PUBLISHING HOUSE
403, Express Tower, Commercial Complex, Azadpur, Delhi-110033 (INDIA)
Phone : 011-27672852 Fax : 91-11-27672046
E-mail : info@satishserial.com, hkjain1975@yahoo.com

ISBN 978-93-81226-29-2

Typeset at: Harminder Singh Kharb *for* Laxmi Art Creation
Printed at: Salasar Imaging Systems, Delhi-110035

Contents

Chapter 1

Exploring Cattle Genome

RAJIB DEB, SUSHIL KUMAR, UMESH SINGH, SANDEEP MANN RANI SINGH AND ARJAVA SHARMA
Project Directorate on Cattle, ICAR, Meerut-250 001, UP, India

Introduction

Domesticated cattle (*Bos taurus* and *Bos taurus indicus*) provide a significant source of nutrition and livelihood to nearly 6.6 billion humans. Cattle belong to a phylogenetically distant clade compared to humans and rodents, known as the Cetartiodactyl order of eutherian mammals, which first appeared 60 million years ago (Murphy *et al.,* 2004). This animal is a representative of the Ruminantia which occupy diverse terrestrial environments with their ability to efficiently convert low quality forage into energy-dense fat, muscle and milk. These biological processes have been exploited by humans since domestication, which began in the Near East some 8,000-10,000 years ago (William 1986). Since then, over 800 cattle breeds have been established representing an important world heritage and an enabling scientific resource for understanding the genetics of complex traits.

As the new genomics era matures, with large-scale genome research and the development of sophisticated bioinformatics tools that can be applied to the agricultural field, agricultural researchers should take advantage of and benefit from new sequencing and mapping technologies. In recent years, the genomes of several domesticated livestock animals have been partially or completely sequenced and especially in past 5-6 years, the functional genomic research field has been revolutionized at unprecedented manner due to the increased application of genome sequencing. Due to the advent of such technologies, it is possible to know the function of various genes, particularly those involved in genetic improvement of animal health and associated with increased food animal production. With the availability of full bovine genomic sequence, it is possible to predict the involvement of specific genes and this in turn helps in improvement of the integrated interactive database (Pareek *et al.,* 2011). Moreover, assembling an individual animal's entire genome sequence or specific region (s) of interest is increasingly important for agricultural researchers to perform genetic comparisons between animals with different performances (Bai *et al.,* 2012). Sequencing of the bovine genome started in December 2003 at the Baylor College of Medicine Sequencing Centre in Houston and is still attaining the status of diversification and versatility. This chapter outlines and discusses about the current status of bovine functional genomics and recent development in bovine genome databases.

Facts Regarding Cattle Genome and Utility of Such Studies

To understand the biology and evolution of ruminants, sequencing of the cattle genome is important. The cattle genome can be assembled with methods similar to the rat and sea urchin genomes and can be used to catalog protein-coding genes, microRNA genes and ruminant-specific interspersed repeats and manually annotated over 4000 genes (Liu *et al.,* 2009). The genome of the animal contains a minimum of 22,000 genes, with a core set of 14,345 orthologs shared among seven mammalian species of which 1,217 are absent or undetected in non-eutherian (marsupial or monotreme) genomes. It has also got transposable element classes similar to other mammals as well as large numbers of ruminant-specific repeats that comprises 27 per cent of its genome. The consensus sequence of BovB, a non-LTR LINE retrotransposon, lacked a functional open reading frame (ORF), suggesting its non-functional nature (Buke *et al.,* 2002). However, BovB repeats with intact ORF have been identified in the genome and their phylogeny indicates that some are still actively expanding and evolving. Cattle-specific evolutionary breakpoint regions in chromosomes have a higher density of segmental duplications, enrichment of repetitive elements, and species-specific variations in genes associated with lactation and immune responsiveness. Genes involved in metabolism are generally highly conserved, although five metabolic genes are deleted or extensively diverged from their human orthologs. Hence, the cattle genome sequence provides an enabling resource for understanding mammalian evolution and accelerating livestock genetic improvement for milk and meat production (Elsik *et al.,* 2009). Moreover, the availability of the bovine genome sequence is useful for both agricultural purposes and human health.

Current Knowledge of Genetic Markers in Bovine

The objective of breeders is to exploit the variability among animals by selecting. The animals with a superior genetic potential for the trait of interest. Many traits suitable for improvement using quantitative genetic methods are easy or inexpensive to measure on a large number of animals whereas many others are not. Several of the meat quality traits are difficult to improve. Such traits include meat tenderness and marbling. Thus, ongoing studies are concentrated on genes that influence genetic potential for these traits to select animals. This is a promising approach because genotyping is now increasingly easy and inexpensive to perform. The advantage of high-throughput techniques of genomics will indeed be the identification and the practical use of polymorphisms within DNA sequences of those genes (Garnier *et al.,* 2003; Barendse 2005). Single nucleotide polymorphisms (SNP) are the most frequent form of DNA variation in mammals. They are abundant, normally biallelic and easy to detect by automatic techniques. So far, polymorphisms in some genes have been reported for their association with tenderness or beef marbling, which is otherwise defined as the amount of visual intramuscular fat (Barendse 2003). They include the genes encoding ú-calpain (Page *et al.,* 2002; White *et al.,* 2005) along with lysyl oxidase and calpastatin (Barendse 2001; Drinkwater *et al.,* 2006) for tenderness.

They also include the genes encoding leptin (Buchanan *et al.,* 2002), DGAT1 (Thaller *et al.,* 2003), TG (Barendse *et al.,* 2004), GH1 (Schlee *et al.,* 1994), SCD, mitochondria (Mannen *et al.,* 1998; 2003), mitochondrial transcription factor A (Jiang *et al.,* 2005) and FABP4 (Michal *et al.,* 2006) for marbling.

Study of Repeat Families and Individual Transposable Elements in Cattle

An examination of repeat families and individual transposable elements within cattle-artiodactyl- and ferungulate-specific evolutionary break point regions (EBRs) have shown a significantly higher density of long interspersed elements-L1 (LINE-L1) elements and the ruminant-specific LINE-RTE repeat family (Kordis and Gubensek 1999) in cattle-specific EBRs relative to the remainder of the cattle genome. In contrast, the short interspersed elements-BovA (SINE-BovA) repeat family and the more ancient tRNAGlu–derived SINE repeats (Shimamura *et al.,* 1997) are present in lower density in cattle-specific EBRs, similar to other long interspersed elements (LINEs) and short interspersed elements (SINEs) (Okada *et al.,* 2004). The differences in repeat densities are generally consistent in cattle-, artiodactyl- and ferungulate-specific EBRs, with the exception of the tRNAGlu–derived and LTR-ERVL repeats, which are at higher densities in artiodactyl EBRs compared to the rest of the genome. The differing density of repeat elements in EBRs were also found in regions of homologous synteny suggesting that repeats may promote evolutionary rearrangements. Differences in repeat density in cattle-specific EBRs are thus unlikely to be caused by the accumulation of repeats in EBRs after such rearrangements occur. A cattle-specific EBR associated with a bidirectional promoter has been identified by researchers that may affect control of the expression of the *CYB5R4* gene which has been implicated in human diabetes and therefore may be important in the regulation of energy flow in cattle. Segmental duplications (SDs) involving genic regions may give rise to new functional paralogs. More than 70 per cent of the cattle SDs correspond to complete or partial gene duplications with high sequence identity. This suggests that many of these gene duplications are specific to either the artiodactyla or the *Bos* lineage and tend to encode proteins that often interface with the external environment, particularly immune proteins and sensory/olfactory receptors. Several of these gene duplications are also duplicated in other mammalian lineages *viz.,* cytochrome P450, sulfotransferase, ribonuclease A, defensins and pregnancy-associated glycoproteins. Paralogs located in segmental duplications present exclusively in cattle may have functional implications for the unique physiology, environment and diet of the animal. An over-representation of genes involved in reproduction in cattle SDs is associated with several gene families expressed in the ruminant placenta. These families encode the intercellular signaling proteins pregnancy associated glycoproteins (on BTA29), trophoblast Kunitz domain proteins (on BTA13) and interferon tau (*IFNT*) (on BTA8). A gene family encoding prolactin-related proteins (on BTA23) is only identified in the assembly-dependent analysis of SDs. These genes regulate ruminant-specific aspects of fetal growth, maternal adaptations to pregnancy and the coordination of parturition (Hashizume *et al.,* 2002). While Type I IFN genes are primarily involved in host defense (Zhang *et al.,* 2008), *IFNT* prevents regression of the corpus luteum during early pregnancy resulting in a uterine environment receptive to early conceptus development (Roberts *et al.,* 2008). Signatures of positive selection that are obtained by measurement of their rates of synonymous and nonsynonymous substitutions haveidentified 71 genes including ten immune related genes (*i.e.IFNAR2, IFNG, CD34, TREM1, TREML1, FCER1A, IL23R, IL24, IL15* and *LEAP2*). As we know, immune genes are over-represented in SDs. Examples of genes varying in cattle relative to mouse include a cluster of â-defensin genes, which encode antimicrobial peptides, the anti-microbial cathelicidin genes (Scocchi *et al.,* 1997), changes in the numbers of interferon genes (Katze *et al.,* 2002) and the number and organization of genes involved in adaptive immune responses in cattle compared to human and mouse. This extensive duplication and divergence of genes involved in innate immunity may be because of the substantial load of microorganisms present in the rumen of cattle which increases the risk of opportunistic infections at mucosal surfaces and positive selection for the traits that enabled stronger and more diversified innate immune responses at these locations. Another possibility is that immunity may have been under selection due to the herd structure which can promote rapid disease transmission.

Approaches in the Detection of Cattle Genome

Cytogenetic analysis of metaphase chromosomes

Cytogenetic analysis of metaphase chromosomes using fluorescence *in situ* hybridization (FISH) allows for the screening of genomic structural variations including Copy Number variations (CNVs). However, these methods have significant limitations both in their resolution that detects structural variations of around 234 Mb. More recently, array comparative genomic hybridization (array CGH) has emerged as a technology that promises to circumvent both of these limitations. These whole-genome arrays are based on long oligonucleotides representing a tiling path along each chromosome. The method has proven successful in detecting hundreds of CNVs. It is possible to assess CNVs and their impact on bovine health in a systematic, cost-effective and high-throughput fashion with the advent of these technologies along with the existence of bovine genome reference sequence (Liu *et al.,* 2008). A set of conservative criteria can be used to define the final set of high confidence CNV calls (Graubert *et al.,* 2007).

Oligonucleotide array

Microarrays of synthetic oligonucleotide probes are becoming increasingly popular for transcriptomic studies in bovine. The power of this approach lies largely in the opportunity to tap into the bovine genome and EST sequencing effort without the need to own libraries that contain probes of interest. Oligo arrays avoid some of the technical errors of cDNA arrays, namely their lack of reliability and spot variability. The reliance on microbiological libraries of clones and their inherent contamination and handling risks has caused problems with reliability for many practitioners. The majority of the variability of microarray spots on cDNA arrays is due to the non-uniform performance of PCR reactions in probe generation. Oligo arrays are therefore of much better quality than cDNA arrays, even in heterologous systems. For example, muscle-specific oligo arrays initially prepared for studies in mice and humans have shown good adaptibility to muscle gene expression studies in cattle (Bernard *et al.,* 2006). A bovine oligo probe set for microarray printing has been marketed by Operon technologies, Inc. market. It is derived from TIGR assemblies of bovine EST and contains about 8,300 bovine genes with a known sequence with a hit to a known human, mouse, or cattle transcript. A bovine long oligo array project has also been developed among a consortium of researchers at Texas A&M University, University of Missouri, Iowa State University, and the University of Minnesota. GenBank sequences are being analysed to remove duplicated sequences, vector sequences and other artefacts of the cloning process. This array has been made available to the international community in 2006 (Elsik *et al.,* 2006). Another oligo array project is currently developed between the University of Illinois, the University of Connecticut and INRA in France. Again, orthologous sequence identification, genomics sequence alignment and insertion deletion analyses were performed for sequence alignment and analysis. Now, coming to the oligonucleotide array construction, genomic DNA can be purified from sperm, whole blood, and ear notch of the animal (Sonstegaard *et al.,* 2008). This technology has been widely used to find out maternal linkage especially in Holstein and Hereford breeds of cattle. Human orthologous gene annotation and overlap can be determined based on net human-cow alignment using the UCSC Genome Browser to find out the relationship status and percentage homologi between cattle and human genome. The microarray for comparative genomic hybridization (CGH) contains 385,048 probes spanning the cattle genome with a median spacing of 5,779 bp. Semen DNA can be tested against Dominette blood DNA or Domino semen DNA and such procedures are especially helpful for detecting DNA copy gains or losses especially in Holstein bull.

Pooled tissue cDNA arrays

Tissue specific microarrays, particularly when they are based on adult tissues, have very clear limitations with respect to discovery of regulatory interactions, as they do not capture the whole transcriptome of the organism. cDNA microarrays with genome-wide representation have therefore been important since many EST collections became available and can be pooled. A bovine cDNA array, known as the

CattleArray 7600 from Pyxis Genomics has become available commercially. Since this array has been made with cDNAs derived from spleen and placenta, it may not be suitable to explore muscle biology and hence beef quality. A number of high-density cDNA arrays constructed for assessing genome-wide gene expression changes in cattle now include genes from muscle-specific libraries. The NBFGC in the USA has selected 18 263 genes from the pooled tissues MARC 1–4 libraries for printing on a high-density microarray (Suchyta *et al.,* 2003). The same strategy has been followed at the Iowa State University where selection of a set of 10,608 EST from MARC 1–4 libraries has been done that include all the known genes and unknown, putative or hypothetical genes expressed in muscle, liver or adipose tissue. The selected genes include 4,484 known genes, 1.170 hypothetical proteins, 497 unknown and 4,364 non-assigned genes. A high-density microarrays based mainly on its collection of immune-specific EST have been developed in United Kingdom (McGuire and Glass 2005). Simultaneously, the company named AgResearch has been using a 10,204 bovine cDNA microarray with broad genome coverage in bovine transcriptome studies (Diez-Tasco´ n *et al.,* 2005).

Clustered SNP genotyping error

Another piece of evidence for the existence of CNVs comes from the bovine SNP data. From the human HapMap data, 1,000 deletion structural variations (1-745 kb) have been discovered by mapping clusters of SNP genotype errors, Mendelian transmission errors along with sites that do not pass Hardy-Weinberg equilibrium (Conrad *et al.,* 2006; Mc Caroll *et al.,* 2006). An initial screen of the first 10,000 SNP data points from cattle has found clustered SNP genotyping errors as candidate deletion variations However, it is evident that the density of SNP markers is too low to achieve a high-resolution map of CNV across the entire genome. These limitations are the critical factors that motivated to continue studying CNV using array CGH.

Utility of Bacterial Artificial Chromosome (BAC) clones for high-quality sequence comparison

Comparison is a fundamental tool for analyzing DNA sequence. Interspecies sequence comparison is particularly powerful for inferring genome function and is based on the simple premise that conserved sequences are likely to be important. Thus, the comparison of a genomic sequence with its orthologous counterpart from another species is increasingly becoming an integral component of genome analysis. In ideal situations, such comparisons are performed with orthologous sequences from multiple species. To facilitate multispecies comparative sequence analysis, a robust and scalable strategy for simultaneously constructing sequence-ready bacterial artificial chromosome (BAC) contig maps from targeted genomic regions has been developed. BAC have been used previously for direct high-quality sequence comparison between breeds like Holstein and Hereford which helps in analysis of large-scale comparative genome that are particularly performed on high-quality finished genomic sequence from cattle, dog, and even humans to study evolutionary changes that have shaped mammalian genomes (Thomas *et al.,* 2002). These same BAC clones from the RP42 library of Holstein breeds have been mapped *in silico* on various versions of the bovine genome assembly. In order to provide high-quality large-scale genomic alignments, the analysis have been mainly limited to the completely finished BAC sequences. Most of these BACs are from the greater cystic fibrosis transmembrane conductance regulator (CFTR) region on bovine chromosome 4, comprising 1.8 Mb of genomic sequence. Insertion/deletion events can be examined in Holstein and Hereford breeds. Ultimately, it gives rise to the fact that SNPs and small indels of size less than 1,000 bp are more common (1 event *i,e.* per 700 bp) by count. However, large-scale events more than 1 kb size are more predominant by length.

Amplified fragment length polymorphism (AFLP) markers for DNA fingerprinting

The AFLP technology produces molecular markers through the high-stringency polymerase chain reaction (PCR)-amplification of restriction fragments that are ligated to synthetic adapters and amplified using primers, complementary to the adapters, which carry selective nucleotides at their 3' ends. In case of cattle, the enzyme combination of *Eco*RI and *Taq*I produces clearer and more polymorphic AFLP patterns. This technique has been used successfully for identifying various polymorphic bands in samples of Italian Holstein genotypes. The number of fragments revealed by each primer combination use to increase significantly the level of genetic information gained in each experiment and the AFLP patterns are reproducible in independent experiments and polymorphic fragments segregate in cattle families according to Mendelian rules (Ajmone-Marsan *et al.,* 2003).

Use of different bead chips for sequencing cattle genome

The Illumina BovineSNP50 is a high-density, genome-wide genotyping array. The v2 Bead Chip contains 54,609 SNPs of major breed types. The probes have been validated in various common beef and dairy breeds. This makes certain types of research, such as QTL discovery and genetic improvement possible (http://www.illumina.com). Although BovineSNP50 have been successfully used, several new chips have also been designed. Besides BovineSNP50 SNPs, Bovine High-Density (HD) Bead Chip of 778K SNP includes some Y-specific and mitochondrial SNPs. Other chips, such as Bovine Low-Density Bead Chip, 96 SNP parentage chip, 384 SNP chip and 700 K SNP Affymetrix chip have also been designed (http://www.slideserve.com).

Bovine HD Bead Chip

The bovine HD Bead Chip is the most comprehensive genome-wide genotyping array that provides superior power to interrogate genetic variation across any breed of beef and dairy cattle. This product has been developed by Illumina in collaboration with major bovine agricultural thought leaders, including USDA-ARS, UNCEIA-INRA, Pfizer Animal Genetics and the University of Missouri. With the advent of this bead chip, over 99 per cent of the markers can be mapped to the UMD3 bovine genome assembly (Zimin *et al.,* 2009), which include coverage of autosomal, mitochondrial and sex-linked (X/Y) SNPs. Uniform genomic coverage, with an average gap size of 3.43 kb and a median gap size of 2.68 kb, provides excellent SNP density to power robust genome-association studies and copy number variation (CNV) detection in cattle (Khatkar *et al.,* 2007). This technology has also lead to the identification and retention of 29,968 loci that appear to have adjacent polymorphism or deletion among the breeds sampled. Although these loci yield lower call rates when compared to most loci on the panel, they can be retained because they may provide biologically relevant information, especially between breed groups (*Bti* vs *Btt*), for traits of interest and future improvements in the genome build. These performance and content validation results clearly demonstrate the robust data quality delivered by the product and such high quality data enables to obtain highest accuracy and reliability for interrogating bovine genotypes in *Bos taurus taurus* and *Bos taurus indicus* breeds. Moreover, there is also availability of Laboratory Information Management System (LIMS) to accurately and efficiently track samples. In addition, robotic automation capabilities can be added to improve throughput for laboratories processing large number of samples. It is also possible to use Illumina's convenient Fast Track genotyping service to have samples genotyped and data delivered in a format suitable for QTL analysis. In nut shell, Bovine HD Bead Chip presents a high-throughput solution for whole-genome studies in any breed of beef and dairy cattle.

Next generation sequencing (NGS) technologies

Next generation sequencing technologies (NGS) using modern platforms to produce significant numbers of sequence fragments have revolutionized research in genetic and biomedical fields and have become increasingly popular in recent years. Several massively parallel platforms are in widespread use by sequencing centers or laboratories at present. These include the Illumina (former Solexa) Genome Analyzer, HiSeq, Roche/454 FLX (http://www.454.com), and the Applied Biosystems Solid System (http://www.appliedbiosystems.com). These platforms can generate millions to billions of reads in a single run with the read length in the range of 50 to 500 bp. The difference between these technologies is embodied in many parameters such as clonal amplification method, instrument as well as sequencing method used and read length generated. Since the number of reads produced and sequencing speed differ among technologies, the generation rate is also different among these technologies. Current Illumina HiSeq technology can generate 150 to 200 Gb data for paired-end 100 bp read length in 8 days. The base call accuracy also varies between these platforms (http:// kevin-gattaca.blogspot.com). Several cutting-edge biological applications such as targeted exome capture or exome sequencing, Chromatin Immunoprecipitation sequencing (ChIP-Seq) and whole transcriptome shotgun sequencing technology, otherwise known as the RNA-Seq have been developed to fulfill different biological purposes. Exome-sequencing (Mamanova *et al.,* 2010) overcomes the drawback of the high cost of sequencing the whole genome by excluding intronic regions and selectively sequencing the exonic regions that might be of more immediate interest. ChIP-Seq (Johnson *et al.,* 2007) is used to identify genome-wide binding patterns of a protein of interest such as a transcription factor and is a powerful approach to study protein-DNA/RNA interactions. RNA-Seq (Mortazavi *et al.,* 2008; Wang *et al.,* 2009) or transcriptome-wide sequencing is used to exploit NGS technologies to sequence cDNAs from RNA samples.

High throughput sequencing of RNA (RNA-Seq) technology

RNA-Seq technology is being used as a popular method for quantitative gene expression studies (Blow 2009) and was primarily developed to analyze global gene expression in different tissues. However, accurate gene expression estimation requires accurate genome annotation (Roberts *et al.,* 2011). By utilizing complete or nearly completely annotated reference genomes, RNA-Seq can assist researchers to identify differentially expressed genes and novel transcripts for agricultural animals in a quantitative and efficient way. The power of RNA-Seq is not only in helping agricultural researchers to select differentially expressed genes between samples under different treatment condition(s) that could be crucial for certain traits or disease resistance, but it can also reveal multiple isoforms that template assembly does not possess in its annotation. There are several popular differential expression testing tools for RNA-Seq data, such as edger (Robinson *et al.,* 2010) and DEGSeq (Wang *et al.,* 2010). Powerful splice junction sites identification tools are represented by Cufflinks (Trapnell *et al.,* 2010)/TopHat (Trapnell *et al.,* 2009) and Supersplat (Bryant *et al.,* 2010). RNA-Seq technology can also assist researchers in annotating transcription of the genome in a complete manner at different developmental stages. Using this specific technology, more than 19,000 genes expressed in milk samples (that accounts for 70 per cent of the total number of genes) have been analyzed. The accuracy of RNA-Seq SNP discovery has been tested by comparing SNPs detected in a set of 42 candidate genes expressed in milk, which have been re-sequenced earlier using Sanger sequencing technology. Seventy of 86 SNPs have been detected using this technology. The validation of unique SNPs, not detected by conventional Sanger's sequencing but found by RNA-Seq, has been done by KASPar genotyping system.Such validation creates guidelines to maximize the accuracy of SNP discovery and prevention of false-positive SNP detection, and provides more than 33,000 SNPs located in coding regions of genes expressed during lactation that can be used to develop genotyping platforms to perform marker-trait association studies, particularly in Holstein cattle (Canovas *et al.,* 2010).

Combination of whole-genome re-sequencing and high-density genotyping arrays

Using a combination of whole-genome re-sequencing and high-density genotyping arrays, genome-wide haplotypes can be reconstructed. More than 1.3 million high-quality SNPs have been detected by such combined technology. The genome-wide haplotypes can be reconstructed using more than 1 million informative SNPs. Comparison of a set of 15,826 SNPs that overlapped in the sequence-based and BovineSNP50 have showed the accuracy of the sequence-based haplotype reconstruction to be as high as 97 per cent. By using the BovineSNP50 genotypes, the frequencies of chief alleles of haplotypes can then be determined in various descendants and the distribution can be compared with the expected frequencies assuming no selection. Around 50 chromosomal segments have already been identified in which chief alleles have shown strong evidence of selection. Candidate polymorphisms for traits that have been under selection in the dairy cattle population have been subsequently identified by referencing DNA sequence within these selected chromosome blocks. Several candidate genes have also been identified with functions related to milk-production, fertility and disease-resistance traits. These data demonstrate that haplotype reconstruction of an ancestral proband by whole-genome re-sequencing in combination with high-density SNP genotyping of descendants can be used for rapid, genome-wide identification of the ancestor's alleles that have been subjected to artificial selection (Larkin *et al.,* 2012).

Combined application of Polymerase chain reaction-Single strand conformation polymorphism (PCR-SSCP) for detection of specific genes in cattle

PCR-SSCP combined technology is found to be especially important for the detection of SNPs of *adiponectin* gene. After detection of the gene, further analysis of the correlation of SNPs with carcass and meat quality traits using the general linear model (GLM) in SPSS program can also be done if PCR-SSCP is performed in a correct manner. Studies have been conducted on several animals of Qinchuan breed to detect five gene types *viz.,AA, AB, BB, CC, CD* with one G>C mutation at 64 bp in exon2 of *adiponectin* in *AB, BB* genetypes and one C->T mutation at 50 bp in exon3 of *adiponectin* in *CD* genetype. It has been found that G->C mutation results in change of glutamic acid (GGA) into glutamine (GCA) and C->T mutation results in change of serine (TCA) into leucine (TTA). Statistical analysis reveals that animal with *AA* genotype is higher than *BB* genotype in slaughter weight, back fat thickness, carcass weight, loin muscle area. The crural girth of *AA* genotype is significantly higher than *AB* and *BB* genotypes. Animals with *CD* genotype is higher than *CC* genotype in slaughter weight, subcutaneous fat thickness, back fat thickness, crural girth and tenderness. *Adiponectin* gene is proved to be closely related to carcass and meat quality traits and such traits can be used as a candidate molecular marker for production of high-grade meat in Qinchuan beef cattle (Jie *et al.,* 2009).

Studies on gene expression profile

The influence of two production systems *viz.,* pasture vs maize silage indoors on muscle gene expression has been studied wherein transcriptomic analyses using a multi-tissue bovine cDNA repertoire have been performed to compare gene expression profiling in rectus abdominis and semitendinosus muscles between both production groups. Variance analysis has shown that the muscle type has an important effect on the expression level of genes (Cassar-Malek *et al.,* 2005).

Before the development of bovine cDNA arrays, human muscle-specific arrays had been used to monitor gene expression throughout development (Sudre *et al.,* 2003). This allows the identification of up to 110 genes differentially expressed from 110 days post-conception to 15 months of age after birth. Among these genes, 33 per cent have unknown functions so far. Most of the differentially expressed genes are either up-regulated or down-regulated at 260 days of foetal development. This confirms the importance of the last three months of gestation in bovine muscle differentiation (Picard *et al.,* 2002).

Muscle hypertrophy is of particular interest in beef meat production as it has a strong economic importance. High muscle development is associated with specific muscle characteristics in favour of only meat tenderness, but not of its flavour. The selection process in favour of muscle growth decreases oxidative muscle activity especially in rectus abdominis which is the most oxidative muscle of both. Some genes are differentially expressed in rectus abdominis and/or semitendinosus between the two groups of bulls with high or low muscle growth potential. Many of them are involved in muscle structure (*e.g.* sarcosin, titin) or in cellular regulation (*e.g.* thyroid hormone receptor interacting protein 10, LEU5, an heat shock protein) and are more expressed in muscles from low muscle growth potential bulls compared to high muscle growth potential bulls (Sudre *et al.,* 2005). Similarly, studies have been conducted in double-muscled (DM) animals which are known to be characterised by a higher muscle mass and a lower fat content in the carcass and in the muscle tissue due to mutation in myostatin which is a negative regulator of skeletal muscle growth which belongs to the transforming growth factor (TGF)-b superfamily. One challenge is nowadays to elucidate the specific mechanisms through which myostatin signals to inhibit the growth of skeletal muscle. About 20 genes have been reported to be differentially expressed between DM and normal-muscled bovine embryos at 31 to 33 days of gestation. These differentially expressed genes fall into general classes including transcription factors, genes involved in protein synthesis and degradation, cell proliferation or altered metabolism. Three of these genes have been physically mapped to bovine chromosome 5, which is very close to a QTL for Warner Bratzler shear force (WBS) at day 14 post mortem and gives an indication of the final toughness of beef. This may be a first step to explain the link between changes in meat tenderness associated with muscle hypertrophy (Potts *et al.,* 2003).

Sequence database of bovine genome

The animal whose DNA was sequenced for the first time is a Hereford cow, named L1 Dominette 0144. The second draft of the bovine genome sequence has been deposited into free public databases. The current assembly named as the Btau 3.0, developed on August 2006, is based on a 7.1-fold coverage of the bovine genome. The sequence data can be accessed via GenBank at NIH's National Centre for Biotechnology Information (NCBI), or via EMBL Bank at the European Molecular Biology Laboratory's Nucleotide Sequence Database and via the DNA Data Bank of Japan. A number of browsers have been developed for the bovine genome: NCBI's Map Viewer, UCSC Genome Browser at the University of California at Santa Cruz, the Ensembl Genome Browser at the Wellcome Trust Sanger Institute in Cambridge, England and the Ruminant-Human Genome Browser at CSIRO, Australia.

Conclusion

Cattle serves as a major source of dairy and meat (*i,e.* protein) for human beings. Genomic research in cattle has to be considered in its different aspects. From the technical point of view, cattle genomics cannot be considered in isolation but will be heavily influenced by the general progress in mammalian genomics. From raw draft assembly to full length cDNA/EST resources and BAC libraries, the cattle population have undergone significant annotations in recent years. The consequence of sequencing the genome of cattle has expanded far beyond the original goals of serving as a model for studying human health issues and physiological phenomena, to increase our understanding of the human genome and to study traits of economic and biological interest to raise cattle production. We are now at the beginning of an era where genome sequencing analysis of cattle allows study of domestication, selection of better breeds having high fertility and understanding of quantitative differences due to environmental factors including nutritional factors.

Gene-gene and gene-environment interactions related to environmental conditions can be studied quantitatively using modern bioinformatics tools. It can clearly be seen that sequencing individual animal genomes or interesting regions under different treatment conditions ultimately benefits the agricultural community by providing guidance for experimental design and animal-disease control and prevention. To summarise, it is expected that the bovine genome sequencing and more generally, any genomic work in cattle will have an impact not only on the livestock industries, but also on all other mammalian research, especially research into human genetics and health.

References

Ajmone-Marsan, P., Vechiotti-Antaldi, G., Bertoni, G., Valentini, A., Cassandro, M. and Kuiper, M. (1997). AFLP markers for DNA fingerprinting in cattle. *Int. Soc. Anim. Genet.,* 28(6): 418-426.

Bai, Y., Sartor, M. and Cavalcoli, J. (2012). Current status and future perspectives for sequencing livestock genomes. *J. Anim. Sci. Biotech.,* 3: 8.

Barendse, W. (2001). DNA markers for meat tenderness. Patent WO02064820.Patent application PCT/AU02/00122. Available: http://ep.espacenet.com/.Accessed: 22 August 2002.

Barendse, W. (2003). DNA markers for marbling. Patent publication WO2004070055. Available: http://ep.espacenet.com/. Accessed: 19 August2004.

Barendse, W. (2005). The transition from quantitative trait loci to diagnostic testin cattle and other livestock. *Australian J. Experiment. Agri.,*45: 831-836.

Barendse, W., Bunch, R., Thomas, M., Armitage, S., Baud, S. and Donaldson, N. (2004). The TG5 thyroglobulin gene test for a marbling quantitative trait locievaluated in feedlot cattle. *Australian J. Experiment. Agri.,* 44: 669-674.

Bernard, C., Cassar-Malek, I., Dubroeucq, H., Renand, G. and Hocquette, J. F. (2006).Gene expression associated with beef sensory qualities. Book of abstracts ofthe 57th annual meeting of the European Association for Animal Production,17–20 September 2006, Antalya, Turkey, p. 46.

Blow, N (2009).Transcriptomics: The digital generation. *Nature.*,458(7235): 239-242.

Bryant, D. W., Shen, R., Priest, H. D., Wong, W. K. and Mockler, T. C. (2010). Supersplat—spliced rna-seq alignment.*Bioinformatics.*,26(12):1500-1505.

Buchanan, F. C., Fitzsimmons, C. J., van Kessel, A. G., Thue, T. D., Winkelman-Sim, D. Cand Schmutz, S. (2002). Association of a missense mutation in the bovine leptingene with carcass fat content and leptin mRNA levels. *Genet. Select.Evol.,* 34: 105-116.

Burke, W. D., Malik, H. S. and Rich, S. M. and Eickbush, T. H. (2002). Ancient lineages of non-LTR retrotransposons in the primitive eukaryotes, *Giardia lamblia. Mol. Biol. Evol.,* 19: 619-630.

Canovas, A., Rincon, G., Islas-Trejo, A., Wickramasinghe, S. and Medrano, J. F. (2010). SNP discovery in the bovine milk transcriptome using RNA-Seq technology. *Mamm. Genome.,* 21(11-12): 592-598.

Cassar-Malek, I., Bernard, C., Jurie, C., Barnola, I., Gente' s, G., Dozias, D., Micol, D.and Hocquette, J. F. (2005). Pasture-based beef production systems may influencemuscle characteristics and gene expression. In Indicators of milk andbeef quality (eds JF Hocquette and S Gigli), EAAP Publication 112, pp. 385-390. Wageningen Academic Publishers, Wageningen, The Netherlands.

Conrad, D. F., Andrews, T. D., Carter, N. P., Hurles, M. E. and Pritchard, J. K. (2006). A high-resolution survey of deletion polymorphism in the human genome. *Nat. Genet.,* 38: 75-81.

Diez-Tasco´ n, C., Keane, O. M., Wilson, T., Zadissa, A., Hyndman, D. L., Baird, D. B., Mc Ewan,J. C and Crawford, A. M. (2005). Microarray analysis of selection lines fromoutbred populations to identify genes involved with nematode parasite resistancein sheep. *Physiol. Genomics.,* 21: 59-69.

Drinkwater, R. D., Li, Y., Lenane, I., Davis, G. P., Shorthose, R. P., Harrison, B. E., Richardson,K., Ferguson, D., Stevenson, R., Renaud, J., Loxton, I., Hawken, R. J., Thomas, M. B.,Newman, S., Hetzel, D. J. S. and Barendse, W. (2006). Detecting quantitative trait lociaffecting beef tenderness on bovine chromosome 7 near calpastatin and lysyloxidase. *Australian J. Experiment.Agri.,* 46: 159-164.

Elsik, C. G., Antoniou, E., Fahrenkrug, S. C., Reecy, J. M., Wolfinger, R. D. and Taylor, J. F. (2006). A bovine whole genome long oligonucleotide expression array. 30[th]international conference on animal genetics, Porto Seguro, Brazil, 20–25August 2006, Abstract C244, p. 68.

Elsik, C. G., Tellam, R. L. and Worley, K. C. (2009). The genome sequence of Taurine cattle: A window to ruminant biology and evolution. *Sci.,* 324(5926): 522-528.

Garnier, J. P., Klont, R. and Plastow, G. (2003). The potential impact of current animalresearch on the meat industry and consumer attitudes towards meat.Meat Sci., 63: 79-88.

Graubert, T. A., Cahan, P., Edwin, D., Selzer, R. R., Richmond, T. A., Eis, P. S. (2007). A high-resolution map ofsegmental DNA copy number variation in the mouse genome. *PLoS.,* 3: e3.

Hashizume, K., Ishiwata, H., Kizaki, K., Yamada, O., Takahashi, T., Imai, K., Patel, O. V., Akagi, S., Shimizu, M., Takahashi, S., Katsuma, S., Shiojima, S., Hirasawa, A., Tsujimoto, G., Todoroki, J. and Izaike, Y. (2002). Implantation and placental development in somatic cell clone recipient cows. *Cloning StemCells.,* 4: 197-209.

http:// kevin-gattaca.blogspot.com.

http://www.appliedbiosystems.com.

http://www.illumina.com.

http://www.slideserve.com.

Jiang, Z. H., Kunej, T., Michal, J. J., Gaskins, C. T., Reeves, J. J., Busboom, J. R., Dovc, P. andWright, R. W. (2005). Significant associations of the mitochondrial transcriptionfactor A promoter polymorphisms with marbling and subcutaneous fat depthin Wagyu £ Limousin F-2 crosses. *Biochem.Biophys. Res.Commun.,* 334: 516-523.

Jie, Y. Y., Linsen, Z. and Hongbao, W. (2009). SNPs detection of *adiponectin* gene and its relationship with carcass and meat quality traits in Qinchuan cattle. 31(10): 1006-1012.

Johnson, D. S., Mortazavi, A., Myers, R. M. and Wold, B. (2007).Genome-wide mapping of in vivo protein-DNA interactions.*Sci.,* 316 (5830): 1497-1502.

Katze, M. G., He, Y. and Gale, M. (2002). Viruses and interferon: a fight for supremacy. *Nat. Rev. Immunol.,* 2: 675-687.

Khatkar, M. S., Zenger, K. R., Hobbs, M., Hawken, R. J. and Cavanagh, J. A. L. (2007). A primary assembly of bovine haplotype block map based on a 15036-single-nucleotide-polymoprhism panel. *Bioinformatics.,* 23(4): 517-519.

Kordis, D. and Gubensek, F. (1999). Molecular evaluation of Bov-B LINEs in vertebrates. *Gen.,* 238: 171-178.

Larkin, D. M., Daetwyler, H. D., Hernandez, A. G., Wright, C. L., Hetrick, L. A., Boucek, L., Bachman, S. L., Band, M. R., Akraiko, T. V., Cohen-Zinder, M., Thimmapuram, J., Macleod, I. M., Harkins, T. T., McCague, J. E., Goddard, M. E., Hayes, B. J. and Lewin, H. A. (2012). *PNAS.,* Edited by: Womack, J. E. (Texas A & M university), College station, TX. doi: 10.1073/ pnas.1114546109.

Liu, G. E., Van Tassell, C. P., Sonstegard, T. S., Li, R. W., Alexander, L. J., Keele, J. W., Matukumalli, L. K., Smith, T. P. and Gasbarre, L. C. (2008). Detection of germline and somatic copy number variations in cattle. *Anim. Genomics Anim. Health. Dev. Biol.,* 132: 231-237.

Liu, Y., Qin, X., Song, X. Z., Jian, H., Shen, Y., Durbin, K. J., Lien, S., Kent, M. P. and Sodeland, M. (2009). Bos taurus genome assembly. *BMCgenomics.,* 10: 180.

Mamanova, L., Coffey, A. J., Scott, C. E., Kozarewa, I., Turner, E. H., Kumar, A., Howard, E., Shendure, J. and Turner, D. J. (2010). Target-enrichment strategies for next-generation sequencing. *Nat. Met.,*7**(2)**:111-118.

Mannen, H., Kojima, T., Oyama, K., Mukai, F., Ishida, T. and Tsuji, S. (1998). Effect ofmitochondrial DNA variation on carcass traits of Japanese Black cattle. *J. Anim. Sci.,* 76: 36-41.

Mannen, H., Morimoto, M., Oyama, K., Mukai, F. and Tsuji, S. (2003). Identificationof mitochondrial DNA substitutions related to meat quality in Japanese Blackcattle. *J. Anim. Sci.,* 81: 68-73.

Mc Carroll, S. A., Hadnott, T. N., Perry, G. H., Sabeti, P. C., Zody, M. C. and Barrett, J. C. (2006). Common deletion polymorphisms in the human genome. *Nat. Genet.,* 38: 86-92.

McGuire, K. and Glass, E. J. (2005). The expanding role of microarrays in the investigationof macrophage responses to pathogens. *Vet. Immunol.Immunopathol.,*105: 259-275.

Michal, J. J., Zhang, Z. W., Gaskins, C. T. and Jiang, Z. (2006). The bovine fatty acidbinding protein 4 gene is significantly associated with marbling and subcutaneousfat depth in Wagyu £ Limousin F2 crosses. *Anim. Genet.,* 37:400-402.

Mortazavi, A., Williams, B. A., Mccue, K., Schaeffer, L. and Wold, B. (2008). Mapping and quantifying mammalian transcriptomes by rna-seq. *Nat. Met.,*5(7): 621-628.

Murphy, W. J., Pevzner, P. A. and O'Brien, S. J. (2004). Mammalian phylogenomics comes of age. *Trends Genet.,* 20: 631-639.

Okada, N., Shedlock, A. M. and Nikaido, M. (2004). Retroposon mapping in molecular systematics. *Met. Mol. Biol.,* 260: 189-226.

Page, B. T., Casas, E., Heaton, M. P., Cullen, N. G., Hyndman, D. L., Morris, C. A., Crawford,A. M., Wheeler, T. L., Koohmaraie, M., Keele, J. W. and Smith, T. P. L. (2002). Evaluation ofsingle-nucleotide polymorphisms in CAPN1 for association with meat tendernessin cattle. *J. Anim. Sci.,* 80: 3077-3085.

Pareek, C. S., Smockzynski, R., Pierzchala, M., Czarnik, U. and Tretyn, A. (2011). From genotype to phenotype in bovine functional genomics. *Briefing in Functional Genomics.,*10(3): 165-171.

Picard, B., Lefaucheur, L., Berri, C. and Duclos, M. J. (2002). Muscle fibre ontogenesisin farm animal species. *Reprod. Nutrition Develop.,* 42: 415-431.

Potts, J. K., Echternkamp, S. E., Smith, T. P. L. and Reecy, J. M. (2003). Characterization ofgene expression in double-muscled and normal-muscled bovine embryos.*Animal Genet.,* 34: 438-444.

Roberts, A., Pimentel, H., Trapnell, C. and Pachter, L. (2011). Identification of novel transcripts in annotated genomes using rna-seq. *Bioinformatics.,*27(17): 2325-2329.

Roberts, R. M., Chen, Y., Ezashi, T. and Walker, A. M. (2008). Interferons and the maternal-conceptus dialog in mammals. *Semin. Sem. Dev. Biol.,* 19: 170-177.

Robinson, M. D., Mc Carthy, D. J. and Smyth, G. K. (2010). Edger: A bioconductor package for differential expression analysis of digital gene expression data.*Bioinformatics.,*26(1): 139-140.

Schlee, P., Graml, R., Rottmann, O. and Pirchner, F. (1994). Influence of growth-hormonegenotypes on breeding values of Simmental bulls. J. Anim. Breeding Genet., 111: 253-256.

Scocchi, M., Wang, S. and Zanetti, M. (1997). Structural organization of the bovine cathelicidin gene family and identification of a novel member. *FEBS.Lett.,* 417: 311-315.

Shimamura, M., Yasue, H., Ohshima, K., Abe, H., Kato, H. and Kishiro, T. (1997). Molecular evidence from retroposons that whales from a clade within even-toed ungulates. *Nature.,* 388: 666-670.

Sonstegard, T. S., Garrett, W. M., Ashwell, M. S., Bennett, G. L., Kappes, S. M. and Van Tassell, C. P. (2000). Comparative mapalignment of BTA27 and HSA4 and 8 to identify conserved segments of genome containing fat deposition QTL. *Mamm. Genome.,* 11: 682-688.

Suchyta, S. P., Sipkovsky, S., Kruska, R., Jeffers, A., McNulty, A., Coussens, M. J., Tempelman,R. J., Halgren, R. J., Saama, P. M., Bauman, D. E., Boisclair, Y. R., Burton, J. L., Collier,R. J., DePeters, E. J., Ferris, T. A., Lucy, M. C., McGuire, M. A., Medrano, J. F., Overton, T. R.,Smith, T. P., Smith, G. W., Sonstegard, T. S., Spain, J. N., Spiers, D. E., Yao, J. and Coussens,P. M. (2003). Development and testing of a high-density cDNA microarrayresource for cattle. *Physiol. Genomics.,* 15: 158-164.

Sudre, K., Cassar-Malek, I., Listrat, A., Ueda, Y., Leroux, C., Jurie, C., Auffray, C.,Renand, G., Martin, P. and Hocquette, J. F. (2005). Biochemical and transcriptomicanalyses of two bovine skeletal muscles in Charolais bulls divergently selectedfor muscle growth. *Meat Sci.,* 70: 267-277.

Sudre, K., Leroux, C., Pie´ tu, G., Cassar-Malek, I., Petit, E., Listrat, A., Auffray, C., Picard,B., Martin, P. and Hocquette, J. F. (2003). Transcriptome analysis of two bovinemuscles during ontogenesis. *J. Biol. Chem.,* 133: 745-756.

Thaller, G., Ku¨ hn, C., Winter, A., Ewald, A., Bellmann, O., Wegner, J., Zu¨ hlke, H.and Fries, R. (2003). DGAT1, a new positional and functional candidategene for intramuscular fat deposition in cattle. *Anim. Genet.,* 34:354-357.

Thomas, J. W., Prasad, A. B., Summers, T. J., Lee-Lin, S. Q., Maduro, V. V. B., Idol, J. R., Ryan, J. F., Thomas, P. J., Mc Dowell, J. C. and Green, E. D. (2002). Parallel construction of orthologous sequence-ready clone contig maps in multiple species. *Genome Res.,* 12: 1277-1285.

Trapnell, C., Williams, B. A., Pertea, G., Mortazavi, A., Kwan, G., van Baren, M. J, Salzberg, S. L., Wold, B. J. and Pachter, L. (2010). Transcript assembly and quantification by rna-seq reveals unannotated transcripts and isoform switching during cell differentiation. *Nat. Biotechnol.*, 28(5): 511-515.

Wang, L., Feng, Z., Wang, X. and Zhang, X. (2010). Degseq: An r package for identifying differentially expressed genes from rna-seq data.*Bioinformatics.*,26(1): 136-138.

Wang, Z., Gerstein, M. and Snyder, M. (2009). Rna-seq: A revolutionary tool for transcriptomics. *Nat. Rev. Genet.,*10 (1): 57-63.

White, S. N., Casas, E., Wheeler, T. L., Shackelford, S. D., Koohmaraie, M., Riley, D. G.,Chase, C. C., Johnson, D. D., Keele, J. W. and Smith, T. P. L. (2005). A new single nucleotidepolymorphisms in CAPN1 extends the current tenderness marker test toinclude cattle of *Bos indicus, Bos taurus*, and crossbred descent. *J. Anim. Sci.,* 83: 2001-2008.

William, R. L. (1986). From husbandry to Science: A highly significient facet of our livestock heritage. *J. Anim. Sci.,* 62: 1742-1758.

Zhang, S. Y., Boisson-Dupuis, S., Chapgier, A., Yang, K., Bustamante, J., Puel, A., Picard, C., Abel, L., Jouanguy, E. and Casanova, J. L. (2008). Inborne errors of interferon (IFN)-mediated immunity in humans: insights into the respective roles of IFN-alpha/beta, IFN-gamma, and IFN-lambda in host defense. *Immunol. Rev.,* 226: 29-40.

Zimin, A. V., Delcher, A. L., Florea, L., Kelley, D. R. and Schatz, M. (2009). A whole genome assembly of domestic cow, *Bos taurus*. *Genome Biol.,* 10(4): R42. 1-10.

□□□

Chapter 2

Hereditary and Congenital Causes of Infertility in Buffalo (*Bubalus bubalis*) Bulls

P. PERUMAL[1], N. SRIVASTAVA[2], M. VEERASELVAM[3], NAZAR SYEDBASHA[4] AND S.K. SRIVASTAVA[2]

[1]NRC on Mithun, Jharnapani, Nagaland – 797 106 [2]IVRI, Izatnagar, Uttar Pradesh – 243 122 [3]Subject Matter Specialist (Animal Science), KVK, Karur, Tamilnadu [4]Research Associate, Animal Physiology Laboratory, NIANP, Bangalore

Introduction

The buffaloes are in the order of *Artiodactyla*, the cloven-hooved mammals, genus *Bubalus* and species *bubalis*. Two main species of buffalo are found in the world: the Asiatic (water) buffalo (*Bubalus bubalis*) and the African buffalo (*Syncerus caffer*). The two buffalo types are have different habitat and chromosome numbers. There are about ~170 million buffaloes in the world. Out of this 97 percent of them are water buffaloes and mainly found in the Asian Region. Riverine buffaloes (70 percent of the total world population) are reared in high numbers in South Asia, especially in India and Pakistan. Swamp buffaloes are found in South-east Asia and Southern China, mainly Thailand, the Philippines, Indonesia, Vietnam, Burma (Myanmar), Laos, Sri Lanka, Kampuchea and.Riverinebuffaloesare predominantly used for milk production and they are also used for meat, fuel and fertilizer production, as well as for draught power, whereas Swampbuffaloesare traditionally kept as draught animals and are also (to a lesser recognition) used for meat production. Improvement of buffalo reproduction helps the production to enhance significantly the economy and living standards of many rural communities throughout the world. The male contributes 50% of germplasm to the herd and is half of the herd. The common defect affects the male fertility are congenital, hormonal imbalance, infectious diseases, hereditary defect, imbalanced nutrition, psychological defect and abnormal climatic condition. In the male animal, fertility can be defined as the ability of a bull to produce semen that will result in a successful pregnancy (Vale, 2009).

Hereditary causes of infertility

The common reproductive problems in buffaloes are late maturity, infertility and sterility (Vale, 2009). Chromosomal abnormalities are one of the causes of lower fertility in cattle and buffaloes (Iannuzzi *et al.*, 2004; Maikinen *et al.*, 2001; Ruvinsky and Spicer, 1999; Iannuzzi *et al.*, 2001; Giovanni *et al.*, 2006; Schepper *et al.*, 1982; Logue, 1978; Rao, 1984; Ahmad *et al.*, 2004; Di Meo *et al.*, 2008; Ansari *et al.*, 1993). Infertility in bulls with apparently excellent semen was traced to intra-chromosomal aberration like translocation and inversion (Gustavsson, 1969). The chromosomal aberration especially the centric fusion has reach high frequencies in bovine population. The famous Robertsonian translocation (1; 29) is found in more than 40 breeds of cattle (Popescu and Pech, 1991) with variable frequencies. In addition to this, various other types of chromosomal abnormalities are reciprocal translocation (Schepper *et al.*, 1982), X- autosome translocation (Basrur *et al.*, 2001), inversion (Popescu, 1990), insertion (Moraes *et al.*, 1987), tandom fusion (Hansen, 1969), balanced autosomal reciprocal translocation (Ansari *et al.*, 1993) and XXY Karyotype with an unusual X; X Translocation (Chauhan *et al.*, 2009). The heritability of various phenotypic and reproductive traits is hardly of 5% or less, which is further compromised by environmental influence (Berglund and Philipson, 2001). Morpho functional disturbance due to hereditary defect are gonadal hypoplasia, epididymal dysfunctions, arrested development of mesonephric ducts, absence or weak libido and it also may be due to inbreeding (Vale, 2009). In buffaloes, chromosomal anomalies involving autosome are translocation (Vijh *et al.*, 1994), chromosomal polymorphism (Patel *et al.*, 1997;Patel and Khoda, 1998), inversions (Balakrishnan *et al.*, 1985), fragile sites (Sanghamitra *et al.,* 2004) and secondary constrictions (Balakrishnan and Yadav, 1984; Patel, 1999) or sex chromosome aneuploidy, such as XO syndrome (Yadav *et al.,* 1990; Prakash *et al.,* 1992; Iannuzzi *et al.,* 2000), XXX syndrome (Balakrishnan and Yadav, 1984; Prakash *et al.,* 1994; Iannuzzi *et al.,* 2004) and XX/XY chimerism (Balakrishnan *et al:,* 1981;Iannuzzi *et al.,* 2005). Sex reversal syndrome (Iannuzzi *et al.,* 2004), XXY-syndrome (Klinefelter's syndrome) with an XX translocation (Patel *et al.,* 2006) and gonadal dysgenesis (Iannuzzi *et al.,* 2001) are also common in this species. The sound neuro-musculo-skeletal system and hoof system is genetically transmittable. Defect such as sickle hocks, post legs and bent or knock knees may affect travel and mounting for mating (Lagerlöf, 1936; Roberts, 1971). Various scrotal configurations are elongated testes, rounded testes, rotated testes, distinctively cleaved testes, testes held too close, unilateral hypoplasia, scrotal hernia and incomplete descent are genetically inheritable and causes infertility to sterility depending on the condition.

Congenital causes of infertility

Congenital anatomical defects of genital organs are due to arrested mesonephric ducts development in the male animals (Vale *et al.,* 2002) are unilateral misplaced testicles, paraphimosis, cryptorchidism, bilateral spermiostasis (Patil and Kaikini, 1972), fusion of ampullae (Chaudhuri *et al.,* 1983), fusion of vesicular gland and unilateral segmental aplasia of wolffian duct (Kaikini and Patel, 1978), under development of seminal vesicle, absence of the testes (Chaudhuri *et al.,* 1983), aplasia of gonads (Kaikini and Patil, 1978), testicular hypoplasia (Kodagali and Bhavasar, 1973; Chaudhuri *et al.,* 1983), bifid scrotum (Kohli and Rajwanshi, 1967; Rao 1980), pseudohermaphroditism, preputial diverticulum (Singh *et al.,* 1986), right unilateral testicular neoplasm (Zanwar, 1974), bilateral testicular aplasia (Arangasamy *et al.,* 2005), testicular aplasia and hypoplasia (Ohashi *et al.,* 1995),congenital umbilical hernia and cryptorchidism (Amle *et al.,* 2004), torsion, displacement and bifid scrotum (Vale *et al.,* 1988, 2009), left testis smaller than the right, with germinal cells absent, tesicular hypoplasia (Vale *et al.,* 2009; Kaikini and Patil, 1978), diphallia (Landy *et al.,* 1986), partial testicular hypoplasia (Ohashi *et al.,* 1988).

The congenital abnormality in buffalo bulls are categorized into three groups

1. Congenital defect of testes
2. Congenital defect of duct system
3. Congenital defect of accessory sex glands

Segmental aplasia of mesonephric duct is most commonly seen in bulls and the body or tail or the entire epididymis may be missing (Blom and Christensen 1951). In majority of the cases, the condition is unilateral and the bulls are sterile and in bilateral cases, the semen is watery with a few or no sperms.

Congenital defect of testes

The common defect testes are testicular aplasia, hypoplasia, absence of testicles, adhesion of tunica vaginalis, under developed testes, bifid scrotum, uni or bi lateral misplaced testes, elongated testes, rounded testes, rotated testes, distinctively cleaved testes, scrotal hernia and incomplete descent of testes. Bulls with abnormalities of testes should not be used for breeding purpose because most of these defects are heritable.

In testicular hypoplasia, there is potential lacking of development of the spermatogenic epithelium and is caused by single recessive autosomal gene with incomplete penetrance with increasing inbreeding (Vale *et al.,* 2009). This is characterized by lack or marked reduction of spermatogenesis in one or both gonads during the fetal life. Testicular hypoplasia is suspected only at puberty or later because of reduced fertility or sterility. The gonadal hypoplasia is a congenital, mostly hereditary condition, which can be unilateral or bilateral and total or partial and unilateral is more common than bilateral (Vale *et al.,* 2009) with the hypoplastic testicle being considerably smaller than that of normally developed and the affected testis to not sink so far down to the bottom of the scrotal pouch. The affected testes are smaller in size about 1/4 to 2/3 of the normal testes (Kaikini and Patil, 1978; Maurya and Bhalla, 1966).

In affected bull, the seminiferous tubules are poorly developed and the reproductive organs are normal because secretion of insufficient testosterone and the animal is poor libido and mounting activity. Histological structure of the hypoplastic testes and epididymis at the head, body and tail has showed that the lumens are lined with low columnar to cuboidal cells with no perceptible micro villi, micropinocytic invagination and eosinophilic bodies. The lumen was devoid of any spermatozoa except for the little fluid or there is presence of high number of immature spermatozoa (9.3%) and low sperm count (650 million per ml) (Arangasamy *et al.,* 2005). In bilateral partial hypoplasia the testis are symmetrical and scrotal circumferences lower than the normal average (Vale 2009). In bilateral segmental aplasia of gonads with fibrous epididymis, the testes are thin, hard, fibrous tissue mass bridging the caput to the corpus epididymis (Kaikini and Patil, 1978).

Congenital defects of Wolffian duct system

Malformation of the male genital / Wolffian duct system are aplasia or hypoplasia of epididymis, epididymal cyst, and cyst of ampullae, epididymitis, spermiostasis, spermatocoel, affection of vas deference and ampullae. It may be unilateral (fertile to infertile) or bilateral (sterile). The epididymis and ampullae segmental aplasia is the most common form of abnormality of Wolffian duct system (Vale *et al.,* 2002). It is characterized by total or partial absence of one or both epididymis and in cattle the right epididymis is common (Chaudhuri *et al.,* 1983). Spermiostasis is caused by blind, rudimentary mesonephric tubules or ductli aberrantis and is probably of genetic origin (Blom and Christensen, 1960).

Congenital defect of accessory glands

The seminal vesicle is one of accessory gland most commonly affected in congenital defect. The congenital defect of the accessory glands is due to developmental abnormalities of the Wolffian duct and hereditary predisposition in the intra uterine life (Luktuke and Namboothiripad, 1977). The common congenital defect are fusion of vesicular gland and unilateral segmental aplasia of seminal vesicles

(Kaikini and Patil, 1978), under development of the seminal vesicle (Chaudhuri *et al.*, 1983), unilateral and bilateral enlargement of the vas deferens, fusion of ampullae (Maurya *et al.*, 1969; Patil and Kaikini, 1972; Kaikini and Patil, 1978), under development of seminal vesicle or cystic vesicle (Luktuke and Namboothiripad, 1977), unilateral segmental constriction of right ampulla (Kaikini and Patil, 1978). The fused ampulla is associated with other genital malformation such as spermiostasis and pigmentation melanosis of the pelvic urethra (Kaikini and Patil, 1978).

Cryptorchidism

Cryptorchidism, or retention of testicles, is commonest type of defective differentiation of the genital system occurring in all domestic species and occasionally in bovines. This condition is sporadic and is due to disordered endocrine secretion. It is due to hereditary defect transmitted by a male and is recessive in bovines. Two or more pairs of recessive genes are involved in many cryptorchid farm animals (Hafez, 2000). Cryptorchid testes are located close to the internal inguinal ring, occasionally may be located under the skin of the ventral caudal abdomen, adjacent to and on either side of the penis, rarely in the femoral canal or in the perineal region. All retained or cryptorchid testes are small, soft and flaccid (Roberts, 1971). The incidence of cryptorchidism in buffalo is rare and is reported in buffaloes. The cryptorchid testicles were located ectopically under the skin of ventral abdomen alongside the penis. The scrotal pouch was found empty (Amle *et al.,* 2004). The retained or cryptorchid testes are usually small in size, soft and flaccid. The retained testes do not produce any spermatozoa (Zanwar, 1974).

Unspecific sperm defects - Dag and Tail Stump Defect

The Dag and Stump tail defect are noticed in exotic breed of cattle especially Jersey and Holstein bulls and are characterized by the presence of high number of unspecific sperm defects with low or absence of motility in the ejaculates (Blom, 1972) and is also reported in Zebu and buffalo cattle (Vale *et al.,* 2009).

Bifid scrotum

In buffalo bulls, common varieties of scrotums are oblong type, square and overlapping types (Somasekaram and Rao, 1986).
Bifid scrotum is due to failure of the scrotal structures at the distal end in buffalo (Rao 1980; Kohli and Rajwanshi, 1967). In bifid scrotum, rotation of scrotum is 90° on its longitudinal axis, separated at the medium phase and are small. The testicles are to be held high up in the scrotum. But the testicles are symmetrical in size and normal in constancy and moved freely with in the scrotal sac. The spermatozoa from such a bulls have high incidence of proximal protoplasmic droplets and semen have a high percentage of abnormal spermatozoa with high head abnormalities (19%) and the most prominent abnormalities present being pear shaped sperms (Rao, 1980).

Preputial diverticulum

Prolapse of prepuce is common in bovine species (Frank, 1981) and the preputial diverticulum is very common in breeding buffalo bulls (Singh *et al.,* 1986) and the symptoms are unable protrude the penis, the swelling enlarge on urination due to accumulation of urine, which will get squeezed due to the pressure of the body while in sitting posture. The preputial diverticulum may be due to forceful thrust of the penis against the preputial fold and leads to swelling and stenosis of the preputial orifice and subsequent development of the diverticulum (Singh *et al.,* 1986).

Congenital defect of external genitalia

Urethral Aplasia

It denotes partial or complete absence of urethra. It is rare condition in male animals. Such condition is usually caused by segmental aplasia of mesonephric duct, which is a genetic defect. The diagnosis can be done by per rectal examination and by semen examination. Prognosis of such condition is poor and treatment is not effective and such males should not be used for breeding purpose (Roberts 1971).

Pigmentation Melanosis

Pigmentation melanosis of pelvic urethra was reported in buffalo male animal (Kaikini and Patil, 1978). The entire urethral mucosa is appear deep dark chocolate brown pigmentation and this condition is associated with other defects such as bilateral segmental gonadal aplasia, bilateral spermiostasis, fusion of ampulla, segmental constriction of ampulla, fusion of vesicular glands (Blom and Christensen, 1972).

Scrotal or inguinal hernia

The hernia depresses the fertility by markedly interfering with the normal thermoregulatory mechanism of the scrotum and testis. It is considered as a common hereditary defect in horses and pigs; less common in bulls, dogs and rams and rare in cats. Scrotal or inguinal hernia causes azoospermia (Raja, 1962) and testicular degeneration (Kodagali, 1977) in buffaloes bulls. Bilateral calcification of testicles is hard and produces grating (metallic) sounds on incision and pin head sized spots of calcification are seen in both testicles (Kaikini and Patil, 1978).

Table 1 : Some cytogenic abnormalities affecting fertility in bovine species

Name of abnormality	Effect	References
Male with trisomy of sex chromosomes and a karyotypes of 61, XXY	Testicular hypoplasia and other disorders	Iannuzzi et al., 2004.
Chromatin mosaicism with cells having 60, XX; 61, XXY and 59, XO karyotypes.	Gonadal hypoplasia, small testes, progeny with reproductive disorders	Maikinen et al., 2001; Ruvinsky and Spicer, 1999.
Translocation between 25th and 27th chromosome in male	Very poor libido and semen of inferior quality	Giovanni et al., 2006.
Translocation between 1 and 29 chromosome in male	Progeny is not fertile	Popescu,1989; Iannuzzi et al., 2001
Translocation between autosome	Low fertility and impaired spermatogenesis	Schepper et al., 1982
Aberrant mitosis	Low conception rate	Logue, 1978
Chromatid linkage	Reduced fertility	Bangso and Basrur, 1976

Break, gap and deletion in X	Sterility	Halnan, 1976.
sex chromosome abnormality: free-martinism	Sterility	Di Meo et al., 2008
XXY chromosome complement with translocation between the two X chromosomes	Sterility	Patel et al., 2006
Balanced autosomal reciprocal translocation	azoospermia	Ansari *et al*., 1993
Translocation	Infertility	Vijh et al., 1994
Chromosomal polymorphism	Sterility	Patel et al., 1997; Patel and Khoda, 1998
Inversions	Infertility	Balakrishnan et al., 1985
Secondary constrictions	Infertility	Balakrishnan and Yadav, 1984; Patel, 1999
XO syndrome	Sterility	Yadav et al., 1990; Prakash et al., 1992; Iannuzzi et al., 2000

Future prospects

The future prospects to improve the reproductive traits and eliminate the reproductive disorders in buffalo bulls are

1. There is a need to greater extent to study sexual development, attainment of puberty, sexual maturity, sex libido, semen production, reproductive performance of buffalo bulls. Study of molecular marker (DNA/gene) assisted selection and cytogenetic studies linked to gene of interest with major effects on reproduction need to be strengthened for selection of breedable male in bubaline species at the early age. This cytogenic marker would help to cull/ eliminate that particular bull from the herd to prevent to spread the genetic/ congenital defective gene from male to future offspring and to prevent reproductive disorders.
2. Breeding soundness evaluation technique would help to improve the breeding efficiency of buffalo bulls.

3. Realistic remedial measures for reducing infertility and enhancing fertility need to be emphasized for the effective control of various reproductive disorders.
4. Biosafety measures for production disease free germ plasm and registration of all A.I. bulls by a national society to initiate a certified disease free semen services for the whole nation need to be addressed.

References

Ahmad, I., Javed, K., Sattar, A. 2004. Screening of breeding bulls of different breeds through karyotyping. Pakistan Veterinary Journal 24(4), 190-192.

Amle, M.B., Shelar, R.R., Thorat, M.G., Zope, A.N. 2004. Congenital umbilical hernia and cryptorchidism in a Pandharpuri buffalo calf. Buffalo Bulletin 23(4), 82-83.

Ansari, H.A., Jung, H.R., Hediger, R., Fries, R., Konig, H., Stranzinger, G. 1993. A balanced autosomal reciprocal translocation in an azoospermic bull.Cytogenetic and Cell Genetics 62, 117-123.

Arangasamy, A., Singh, R., Singh, L.P., 2005: Bilateral aplastic testes in adult buffalo bull (*Bubalus bubalis*). Indian J Anim Reprod 26(2), 174-175.

Arthur, G.H., Noakes, D.E., Pearson, H. 1989. Veterinary Reproduction and Obstetrics, 6th ed., ELBS, Bailliere Tindall, London.pp. 509, 551.

Balakrishnan, C.R., Yadav, B.R. 1984. Normal and abnormal chromosomes in the Indian river buffalo. Buffalo Bulletin3, 13-17.

Balakrishnan, C.R., Yadav, B.R., Sharma, P.A., Goswami, S.L. 1981. Sex chromosome chimerism in heterosexual Murrah buffalo triplets.Veterinary Record109, 112.

Balakrishnan, C.R., Yadav, B.R., Sharma, P.A., Yadav, J.S. 1985. Spontaneous pericentric inversion in Indian buffalo *Bubalusbubalis*.The Nucleus28, 45-48.

Basrur, P.K., Reyes, E.R., Farazmand, A., King, W.A., Popescu, P.C. 2001. X-Chromosome translocation and low fertility in a family of crossbred cattle.Animal Reproduction Science 67, 1-16.

Berglund, B., Philipson, J. 2001. Breeding for dairy cattle fertility – the Scandinavian experience.Proceedings of the Reproductive Failure in Farm Animals Symposium pp. 5-11.

Blom, E. 1976.A sterilizing "tail stump sperm defect" in a Holstein Friesian bull.Norden Veterinary Medicine 28, 295-298.

Blom, E., Christensen , N.O. 1972. A systematic search for abnormalities in testis- epididymis in pedigree bulls in Denmark. Studies on pathological condition in the testis, epididymis and accessory glands in the bulls.Year book, Royal Vet.andAgric. College, Copenhagen, pp. 1-36.

Blom, E., Christensen, N.O. 1960. The etiology of spermiostasis in the bull.Studies on pathological conditions in the testis, epididymis, and accessory glands in the bull.V Nord Veterinaermed 12, 453-470.

Chaudhuri, N., Purbey, L.N., Parihar, N.S. 1983. Studies on the abnormalities of vas deferens, ampulla and seminal vesicles in non- descript buffalo. Indian Journal of Animal Health 22, 15-19.

Chauhan, J.B., Patel, R.K., Singh, K.M., Soni, K.J. 2009. Impact of a novel cytogenetic finding (unusual X;X translocation) on fertility of a buffalo bull (*Bubalusbubalis*). Buffalo Bulletin 28 (3), 151-153.

Di Meo, G.P., Perucatti, A., Di Palo, R., Iannuzzi, A., Ciotola, F., Peretti, V., Neglia, G., Campanile, G., Zicarelli, L., Iannuzzi, L. 2008. Sex chromosome abnormalities and sterility in river buffalo. Cytogenetic and Genome Research 120 (1-2), 127-31.

Frank, E.R. 1981. Veterinary surgery.1st Indian edition.GBS Publisher. New Delhi. pp.300-302.

Giovanni, A., Incarnato, D., Guedes-Pinto, H., Eggen, A., Iannuzzi, L. 2006. Cattle rob (1;29) originating from complex chromosome rearrangements as revealed by both banding and FISH mapping techniques. Chromosome research 154(6), 649-655.

Gustavsson, I. 1969. Cytogenetics, distribution and phenotypic effects of a translocation in Swedish cattle. Hereditas 63, 68 – 169.

Hafez, B., Hafez, E.S.E. 2000. Reproduction in Farm Animals, 7th ed., Lippincott Williams and Wilkins, Philadelphia pp.279-281, 313.

Hansen, K.M. 1969. Bovine tandem fusion and fertility.Hereditas 63, 453-454.

Iannuzzi, L., Di Meo, G.P., Perucatti, A., Zicarelli, L. 2000. A case of sex chromosome monosomy (2n = 49, X) in the river buffalo (*Bubalus bubalis*). Veterinary Record147, 690-691.

Iannuzzi, L., Di Meo, G.P., Perucatti, A., Ciotola, F., Incarnato, D., Di Palo, R., Peretti, V., Campanile, G., Zicarelli, L. 2005. Freemartinism in river buffalo: clinical and cytogenetic observations. Cytogenetics and Genomic Research108, 355-358.

Iannuzzi, L., Di Meo, G.P., Perucatti, A., Di Palo, R., Zicarelli, L. 2001. 50, XY gonadal dysgenesis (Swier's syndrome) in a female river buffalo (*Bubalusbubalus*). Veterinary Record 148, 634-635.

Iannuzzi, L., Di Meo, G.P., Perucatti, A., Incarnato, D., Di Palo, R., Zicarelli, L. 2004. Reproductive disturbances and sex chromosome abnormalities in river buffaloes. Veterinary Record 154, 823-824.

Jones, T.C., Hunt, R.D. 1983.Congenital lesions of the cerebellum. In: Veterinary Pathology, Jones TC, Hunt RD, 5th ed., Lea and Febiger, Philadelphia. pp. 1656–1660.

Kaikini, A.S., Patil, R.K. 1978. Studies on genital malformation of Berari (Nagpuri) buffalo bulls. Indian Journal of Animal Science 48,411-413.

Kodagali, S.B. 1977. Precedings of 1st All India Symposium of Animal Reproduction. Ludhiana, India.

Kohli, I.S., Rajwanshi, D.S. 1967. A case of bifid scrotum in a buffalo bull. Indian Veterinary Journal 44, 257.

Lagerlöf, N. 1936.Sterility in bulls.Veterinary Record 48, 1159-1170.

Landy, B., Signer, R.andOetjen, L. 1986. A case of diphallia. Urology 28(1), 48-49.

Logue, D.N. 1978. Meiosis and spermatogenesis in bulls heterozygous for a presumptive 1/29 Robertsonian translocation.Journal of Reproduction and Fertility 54, 159.

Luktuke, S.N., Namboothiripad, T.R.B. 1977. Journal of Remount Veterinary Corps 16, 45-57.

Maikinen, A., Suojala, L., Niini, T., Katila, T., Katila, T., Miyak, Y.I., Hasregawa, T.2001. X- Chromosome detection in a XO mare using a human X paint probe, and PCR detection of SRY and amelogenin genes in 3 XY mares. Equine Veterinary Journal 33, 527:530.

Maurya, S.N., Bhalla, R.C. 1969. Review: Testicular hypoplasia in buffalo bulls. Indian Veterinary Journal 43, 669.

Moraes, J.C.F., Mattevim, S., Silva, J.F. 1987. Fertility effects of chromosomes rearrangement (insertion 16) in Charolais cattle from Brazil. Theriogenology 27, 665 – 678.

Ohashi OM, Vale WG, Sousa JS, Silva AOA, 1995: Distrubance of testicular development in buffaloes (*Bubalus bubalis*): hypoplasia and aplasia. Buffalo J 11, 97-101.

Ohashi OM, Sousa JS, Vale WG, 1988: Aspecto reprodutivo no macho bubalino. In: Bubalinos: fisiologia e Patologia da Reprodução. Fundação Cargill, São Paulo. pp.69-86 (cited from Vale WG, 2007: Effects of environment on buffalo Reproduction. Ital J Anim Sci 6 (Suppl. 2), 130-142).

Patel, R.K. 1999. Presence of unusual secondary constrictions in smallest autosome of subfertile Murrah buffalo bull (*Bubalus bubalis*). Buffalo News Letters 12, 4-7.

Patel, R.K., Khoda, V.K. 1998. Presence of variant chromosome 3 in the infertile water buffaloes (*Bubalus bubalis*). Veterinary Review13, 25-27.

Patel, R.K., Radhakrishna, U., Khoda, V.K. 1997. Mitotic disturbances associated with variant chromosome 3 in river buffalo bulls (*Bubalusbubalis*). Buffalo Journal 2, 173- 178.

Patel, R.K., Singh, K.M., Soni, K.J., Chauhan, J.B. 2006. Noval cytogenetic finding: an unusual X; X translocation in Mehsana buffalo (*Bubalus bubalis*). Cytogenetics and Genomic Research 115, 186-188.

Patil, R.K., Kaikini, A.S. 1972. Studies on certain aspects of reproduction in Berrri (Nagpur) buffalo bulls. In: FAO Swedish fellow-up seminar on animal reproduction, vol.1 Bangalore, India.

Popescu, C.P., Pech, A. 1991. Une bibiliographie sur la translocation 1/29 de bovines dans le monde (1964 – 1990). Annales De Zootechnie 40, 271-305.

Popescu, P.C. 1990. Consequences of abnormalities of chromosome stricture in demostic animal. Reproduction Nutrition Devevelopment Supplement 1, 105-116.

Prakash, B., Balain, D.S., Lathwal, S.S. 1992. A 49, XO sterile Murrah buffalo (*Bubalus bubalis*).Veterinary Record130, 559-560.

Prakash, B., Balain, D.S., Lathwal, S.S., Malik, R.K. 1994. Trisomy -X in a sterile river buffalo. Veterinary Record134, 241-242.

Raja, C.K.S.V. 1962.Azoospermia in a breeding bull.Kerala Veterinary Journal 3, 107.

Rao, A.R. 1980. A case of bifid scrotum associated with mild disturbances in spermatogenesis. Indian Veterinary Journal 57, 1041.

Rao, A.R. 1984. Proceeding of 10th International Congress.Animal Reproduction Science 25, 109-113.

Ribeiro, H.F.L., Vale, W.G. 2007. Dag defect in Murrah buffalo bulls in Brazil. Italian Journal of Animal Science 6 (2), 667-670.

Roberts, S.J. 1971. Veterinary Obstetrics and Genital Diseases, 2nd ed., CBS Publishers India. pp. 47, 54, 664-665.

Ruvinsky, A., Spicer, L.J. 1999. Developmental genetics. In "The Genetics of Cattle", (Fries R, Ruvinsky A, eds), CABI Publishing and CAB International, Wallingford, Oxon, UK.

Sane, C.R., Kaikini, A.S., Luktuke, S.N., Hukeri, V.B., Deshpande, B.R., Velhankar, D.P., Kodagali, S.B., Deopurkar, V.L. 1994.Reproduction in Farm Animals, Second ed., Verghese Publishing House, Mumbai, pp.133.

Sanghamitra, K., Patel, R.K., Sambasiva Rao, K.R.S., Singh, K.M. 2004. Preliminary study on detection of fragile site on chromosomes of sub-fertile Murrah buffalo bull. Haryana Veterinarian 43, 68-71.

Schepper, G.G., Aalbers, J.G., Brake, J.H.A. 1982. Double reciprocal translocation heterozygosity in a bull.Veterinary Record110, 197- 199.

Singh, S.S., Pradad, B., Sharma, S.N., Ramkumar, R. 1986. Preputial diverticulum in a buffalo bull. Indian Veterinary Journal 63, 693.

Somasekaram, G., Rao, A.R. 1986. Different types of scrotii and their relationship with semen charactertics of murrah buffalo bulls. Indian Journal of Animal Reproduction **7**:124.

Vale, W.G. 2009. Genetic and Environmental Influence on Breeding Performance of Brazilian Buffalo Bulls. Pakistan Journal of Zoology 9, 467-477.

Vale, W.G., Silva, A.O.A., Sousa, J.S., Pereira, W.L.A., Magalhaes, A.N., Oliveira, C.M.C., Ribeiro, H.F.L. 2002. Arrested development of the mesonephric ducts in a Murrah buffalo bull.1st Buffalo Symposium of Americas.pp. 479-481 (Abtr.).

Vijh, R.K., Tanita, M.S., Sahai, R. 1994. Translocation in Murrah buffalo.Indian Journal of Animal Science 64, 534-538.

Yadav, B.R., Kumar, P., Tomar, O.S., Kumar, S., Balain, D.S. 1990. Monosomy X and gonadal dysgenesis in a buffalo heifer (*Bubalus bubalis*). Theriogenology34, 99-105.

Zanwar, S.G. 1974. M.V.Sc. Thesis Konkan Krishi Vidyapeeth, Dapoli, India (cited from Rao AR, 1997: Reproductive disorders in Indian livestock, 1st edition Revised, ICAR, New Delhi, pp. 136).

□□□

Chapter 3

Transgenic Animals and its Applications

P. PERUMAL[1], J.K. CHAMUAH[1], GOKULDAS P.P[2]., E.M. SADEESH[3]
[1] NRC on Mithun (ICAR), Jharnapani, Nagaland
[2] NRC on Pig (ICAR), Rani, Guwahati, Assam [3]CIRB (ICAR), Hisar, Hissar, Haryana

Introduction

The discovery of genetic code about 40 years ago suggested that the gene isolation and transfer in to living organism would become major tool for biologist. The first gene transfer into mouse using isolated DNA revealed that the generation of animals stably harboring foreign DNA (Gordon *et al.,* 1980) with modified phenotypic characters (Palmiter *et al.,* 1982) was made. These pioneer and fascinating experiment also revealed some of the limits of transgenesis, the generation of transgenic animals by gene microinjection appeared laborious. It is now well established that transgenesis is one of the major tool of the biologist to study gene expression and function. Transgenesis is still going to be used more extensively and systematically with the identification of all human genes. Transgenesis also play an essential role for application in the medical and agronomic fields. The study of human diseases is greatly facilitated by the generation of transgenic animals mimicking health disorders of allowing the evaluation of the new pharmaceuticals interest, one being prepared in the milk as transgenic animals. A few lines or farm animals having improved breeding properties have been generated and are understudy for human consumption. Despite the impressive and growing success, transgenesis still suffers from many imperfections.

Transgenic Construction and Design

The original definition described a transgenic animal as one carrying recombinant DNA molecules that was introduced by intentional human intervention (Gordon and Ruddle, 1981). Transgenesis defined as the introduction of foreign DNA sequence in the genome of multicellular organism and ensuring that the sequences are transmitted to the progeny of the manipulated species (Houdebine, 2003). On the other hand, Brink *et al.,* (2000) defined as alteration of the genetic information with the intention as modifying a physical charactertics of animals. Transgenesis differs from the gene therapy since the farmer; the inserted gene is exported to be transmitted to the next generation but in gene therapy, the gene will not be transmitted to next generation. Furthermore, the term transgenic has wider implications since it could compromise animals which had additional (knock in) or deletion (knock out) of genes from the genome.

A transgene is a recombinant DNA molecule that includes two parts regulatory element and structural element. The regulatory element confers tissue specificity and controls when the gene expression during development and modulates the amount of gene expression. The structural element is composed of DNA sequence that encodes the genetic information needed to synthesis the gene product (Wall*et al.,* 1997). The regulatory element includes promoter, enhancer, silencer, insulator element locus control region (LCR), introns and poly - A sequence. The selection of transgene, which should be based on the economic, scientific and social realities. The transgene which codes for the protein of interest can be derived from another animal of the same species, from a different species, even from the bacteria or plants. The regulatory element should be chosen such a way that enhance or enable control of gene expression (Wiqmann and Kues, 2003).

Methods to generate transgenic animals

During the past decades various methods have been developed to generate the transgenic animals. With the advent of gene sequencing many sequences have been determined bringing the knowledge of promoters and gene of interest for various species. The advent of genomics, proteomics and the new generation of reproductive biotechnologies hold the promise of successful application as transgenesis to domestic animals (Collores *et al.,* 2005).

The techniques and methodologies to be implemented in the generation of the transgenic animal depend upon the targeted use of the animals.

Transgenic animals have been produced by a number of techniques

- Pronuclear microinjection
- Nuclear transfer
- Retroviral mediated gene transfer
- Lentiviral mediated gene transfer
- Sperm mediated gene transfer
- Testis mediated gene transfer
- Transposon mediated gene transfer
- Artificial chromosome mediated gene transfer

Applications of Transgenesis

Livestock production

Enhanced prolificacy and reproductive performance increased feed utilization and growth rate, improved carcass consumption, improved milk production or composition and increased disease resistance are practical application of transgenesis.

Modification of milk

Advances in recombinant DNA technology have provided the opportunity to change the composition of milk, increase in milk volume and to produce entirely novel proteins in milk. These changes may add value, as well as increase the partial uses of milk. Clearly altering the charactertics of one of the components to enhance a particular processing feature may make milk unsuitable for other uses. Many of proposed changes in milk structures are listed in table 1.

S.No.	Changes	Consequences
1.	Increase α and β- CN	Enhanced curd firmness for cheese making, improved thermal stability and increased calcium content
2.	Increase phosphorylation site in caseins	Increased calcium content and improved emulsification
3.	Introduce proteolytic sites in caseins	Increased rate of texture development (improved cheese ripening)
4.	Increases α CN concentration	Enhanced stability of casein aggregates, decreased micelle size and gelation and coagulation
5.	Eliminates β- LG	Decreased high temperature gelation, improved digestibility, decreased allergenic response and decreased primary source of cystein in milk.
6.	Decrease α - LA	Decreased lactose, increased market potential of fluid milk, decreased ice crystal formation and compromised osmotic regulation of mammary glands
7.	Add human lactoferrin	Enhanced iron absorption and protected against gut infection
8.	Add proteolytic sites to α-CN	Decrease rate of cheese ripening
9.	Decrease expression of acetyl carcaboxylase	Decreased fat content, improved nutritional quality and reduced milk production cost
10	Express Ig genes	Protected against pathogens such as salmonella and listeria
11	Replace bovine milk proteins gene with human equivalents	Mimicked human breast milk

Transgenic pigs containing the bovine alpha lactalbumin (α-LA) gene, which improve milk production and composition in swine. Alpha lactalbumin is a component of lactose synthesis complex and is involved in the synthesis of lactose in milk (Bleck *et al.,* 1998). Furthermore, higher concentration of α - LA early in the lactation boost milk output and piglet growth. In fact, piglet growth rate is higher when the piglet are sucking sow contain the a-LA transgenic. It has been suggested that bioactive substances (IGF, TGF- α and lactoferrin) in the milk possess important function in the neonate. These proteins influence growth as well as development and maturation of the gut, the immuno system and the endocrine organs (Grossvenor *et al.,* 1993). The over expression of a number of these proteins in milk through the use of the transgenic animals may improve the growth, development, health and survivability of the developing offspring.

Modification of growth and carcass composition

Introduction of porcine growth hormone (PGH) genes into swine genome increases the growth rate, without increased arthritis and abnormal skeletal growth (Vise *et al.,* 1988). An alternative approach was performed hypertrophy of numerous muscles while reducing body fat by introduction of the chicken ski mutant oncogene, which was previously shown to cause (Sutrave *et al.,* 1990). This strategy, however, has resulted in limited success although muscle hypertrophy has been observed in some transgenic pig and transgenic cattle (Bowen *et al.,* 1994). The myostatin (growth differentiation factor-8, GDF-8) gene normally present in mouse skeletal muscle. Myostatin serves as autocrine prenatal inhibitor of myoblast differentiation and growth, when it knocks out result in an increase in lean muscle mass (McPherron *et al.,* 1997). Such genes also present in livestock hence same approaches can be used made in livestock to improve their lean muscle production.

Modification of disease resistance

Identification of single gene in the major histocompatibility complex (MCH), which influences the immune responses, was instrumental in the reorganization up genetic basis of disease resistance or susceptibility. It has only been realized recently that there are many aspects of disease resistance or susceptibility in livestock that are genetically determined (Lewin, 1989).manipulation of the MCH in farm animal through ES cell or NT transgenesis could have a major beneficial effect on disease resistance for livestock producers.

Mice and mouse fibroblast cell line that contain the Mx protein were shown to be resistant to infection with influenza virus (Haller *et al.,* 1981). The Mx cDNA has been introduced into porcine fertilized ova, producing pigs that are resistant to influenza infection (Muller *et al.,* 1992).

Prion is infectious agent that causes spongiform encephalopathies in human and animals. PrP^c or the normal protein is expressed in outer surface of neurons. A switch causes the prion disease from the normal PrP^c to a modified form of PrP. Bueler et al. (1993) demonstrated the inactivation of gene by homologous recombination in mice and this mouse is resistant to spongiform encephalopathy. The same knocking out can be done in sheep and cattle to improve the disease resistance to scrapie and bovine spongiform encephalitis. The antibacterial proteins such as lysostaphin can be used to confer resistance to bovine mammary gland infection. This protein has potent antistaphylococcal activity and its secretion into milk conferred substantial resistance to infection in three lines of transgenic mice (Kerr and Wellnitz, 2003).

Modification of wool production

Alteration of the protein composition of wool fiber via transgenesis with sheep wool keratin and keratin associated protein (KAP) gene may lead to the production of fiber types with improved processing and wearing qualities (Bawden *et al.,* 1998). These authors obtained wool fibers with higher luster and reduced crimp as a result to alteration in their micro and macro structure due to a high level of cortical specific expression of a wool type II intermediate filament (f) keratin gene.

Modification of digestion

Phytase is an enzyme that cleaves inorganic phosphorous form to organic form which increases the phosphorous availability to the animals. This enzyme normally presents in ruminates but absent in monogastric animal. By additional supply of this enzyme along with feed make better utilization of feed (Umadevi, 2006). Golovan et al. (2001) produced the transgenic pig which expresses the phytase enzyme in their saliva, which enhance the digestion and reduce the feed cost in pig production.

Application as bioreactor

The production of therapeutic proteins represents the first application of recombinant DNA technology, by the 2003; the European Union had approved 88 products. However none of this approved product was obtained in transgenic system. Despite this, domestic animals represent on efficient production system for large and complex (and biologically active) recombinant protein, which would be used to treat or prevent human disease. The production of these pharmaceutical proteins in the mammary gland of livestock originated the term biopharming (Keefer, 2004) or gene pharming (Wall, 1999). Various investigators have produced transgenic rabbit, sheep, goat, pig and cattle express heterologous protein successfully. The production of biopharmaceuticals present the most varied purposes: for treating such disease as multiple sclerosis, hepatitis, cystic fibrosis, blood disorders, some type of cancers, haemophilia, thrombosis, growth disorders, pompe's disease, osteoporosis, Paget's disease and anemia and for improving infant's formula.

Initially the use of transgenic animals as bioreactors focused on the use of mammary glands as target but today blood, bladder, eggs and male accessory glands have all have been considered as bioreactors for pharmaceutical proteins.

Transgenic mammary glands

1. Advantages of pharmaceutical proteins expressed in milk include
2. The mammary gland is a prodigious production system that is cable of generating between 23 gm (dairy cattle) and 205 gm (rat) of protein / kg of body weight during peak lactation (Oftedal, 1984).
3. Milk is clearly the least complicated body fluid to collect especially from ruminants.

4. Another advantage of producing biologically active products using the mammary gland is the isolation of the mammary gland from circulatory system. It is argued that bioreactor animals would be protected from the potentially untoward effect of biologically active compound because those compounds would be sequestered in the mammary gland and there fore would be unavoidable to the circulatory system.
5. Proteins which are expressed through mammary gland are able to post translation modification and also biologically active.

Human milk lysozyme is an important protein for innate immunity, but human breast milk is a fairly poor source of commercial production of this enzyme. Lysozyme is one of the most important antibacterial factors in milk, because it hydrolyzes the glycoside β linkage between N-acetylmuramic acid and N acetylglucosamine acid of the peptidoglycan polymer in the bacterial cell wall (Imoto *et al.*, 1972). Milk lysozyme has three times more lytic activity than that of egg white lysozyme because it possesses a greater positive charge than latter (Parry *et al.*, 1969). Lysozyme, which helps to increase the level of beneficial microorganism in the infants and strength of their disease resistance. Li *et al.*, 2006 successfully expressed the human lysozyme in the milk of transgenic mice and also it is biologically active. It can be express in cows milk that with helpful to create disease resistance in many orphan child.

Limonta et al. (1995) produced the transgenic rabbit for production of human growth hormone using whey acid protein gene promotor. The growth hormone enhances the growth retarded children. Recombinant pig growth hormone causes a massive in muscle mass (Evock *et al.*, 1988) hence it also used for increase the body weight in pig.

Lactoferrin present in human milk is an iron binding glycoprotein, which has bacteriostatic and bactericidal effect on the gram positive and gram negative bacteria. This helps to prevent bacterial infections that cause digestive problem that harm or kill millions of newborns around the world. Now transgenic bull was developed for human lactoferrin gene and it was named as Herman. Herman has now fathered for many calves (Pursel, 1995). Herman is produced by gene pharming Europe, B.V. Company (Netherlands).

Breathed air contains many living organism where it enters the lungs. The lungs contain large numbers of neutrophils. These neutrophils secrete elastase and clear the organism. The walls of the alveoli in the lungs contain elastin, which maintains the elasticity of the lungs and this can be also be broken down by elastase and cause emphysema of the lung. To prevent this from happening there is secreted into the blood serum an enzyme called α 1- protease inhibitor (previously called α1-antitrypsin) or α PI. Now this 1- antitrypsin successfully expressed in transgenic sheep and it named as Tracy grazes by PPL therapeutic company (UK). That can be purified and used for treatment of emphysema of lung (Pursel, 1995).

Several companies are developing protein therapeutics produced in milk. GTC biotherapeutics, C1 inhibitor for treatment of hereditary angio-oedema, produced in transgenic rabbit milk by pharming group N.V.

Biosteel is an extra ordinary new product that may soon be used in bullet proof vests and in suture silk for closing up of wounds. Fundamentally biosteel is spider web, which is among the strongest fiber on the earth. The gene of spider silk has been successfully transferred into goat by nexia biotechnologies (Canada) and those goat's milk contains the protein that make up spider silk (Thiemann *et al.*, 2004).

In 1997, Polly is the transgenic sheep that express the human blood clotting factor IX in their milk. It is produced by nuclear transfer technique. Human antithrombin – III (AT- III) is normally presents in human blood and it prevents clotting in the veins. Some people with an inherited deficiency (lack) of this protein are more prone to blood clots, which are dangerous when they break free lodge in lung or brain. To prevent this that patient need to take repeated injection at AT- III. Now Genzyme Corporation company and also produced AT – III producing goat farm successfully express it in goat milk.

A variety of human have been expressed in milk of several species of animal including insulin like growth factors I in rabbit, α - lactalbumin in cows and protein C in pig (Rudolph, 1999). The enzyme α-glucosidase from the milk of transgenic rabbit has been successfully used for by treatment of pompe's disease in infants (Hout, 2004).

The animal of choice for expression of foreign gene in milk is rabbit because of early age of maturity, short gestation period and multiparous than the other farm animals.

Transgenic urinary bladder

Kerr *et al.* (1998) successfully expressed the human growth hormone in the transgenic mouse bladder epithelium using a promotor of mouse Uroplakin II gene.

There are some advantage in expressing in urine are

1. We can use both male and female animals
2. Non invasive collection of product
3. Ability to harvest product shortly after birth from both sexes

Transgenic blood

Swanson et al. (1992) successfully expressed the human haemoglobin in transgenic swine blood. This hemoglobin could be purified from their blood and used to create a blood substitute to give to human patient because pigs are so easy to breed, they could provide an unlimited supply of inexpensive hemoglobin. This supply could help to solve the problem of blood shortages.

Transgenic seminal vesicle

Dyck et al. (1999) expressed the human growth hormone in transgenic mice seminal vesicle using a mouse P_{12} gene promotor. The concentration they obtained is 0.5 mg/ ml. it is prove to be an alternative to use of the mammary gland as a bioreactor. The animal of choice for this type of expression is boar, because their ejaculates 200-300 ml/ ejaculation with a total protein 30 mg/ml and can ejaculate 2-3 times per week, year round (Setchell, 1988). Therefore, a single transgenic pig expressing of foreign protein under the control of a similar promotor specific to accessory sex gland at a rate of 1.0 mg/ml could produce 22.4gm of protein/ year.

Transgenic eggs

Eggs are inexpensive source at high quality protein, but many people avoid them because they are rich in cholesterol. Altering the gene responsible for cholesterol production could result in healthier, lower cholesterol eggs. Low cholesterol eggs food that could help to produce many health problems in peoples (Thiemann *et al.,* 2004). Recently chicken anti-Prion single chain antibody expressed successfully in transgenic quail eggs using β actin promotor. They also checked their biological activity of that protein using western blotting analysis (Kawabe *et al.,* 2006).

Application in xenotransplantation

The demand of organ transplantation is much greater than the supply of organ from human donors. It is estimated that every year, 10 -15 % patients in United States die while waiting for heart or liver donors (Logan, 2000). Pigs are primary interest for organ donation because their physiology and other parameters, including organ size, indicate that they are the among the most suitable non primate potential donor species. The major antigen that stimulate hyper acute rejection is the $\alpha_{1,3}$ – galactose ($\alpha_{1,3}$ Gal) epitope, which is found on the organ and secreted glycoprotein of all mammals except in humans, apes and old world monkeys (Sachs *et al.,* 2001). This epitope is synthesized by the enzyme $\alpha_{1,3}$ galactosyl transferase ($\alpha_{1,3}$ – GT), but the enzyme is inactive in humans. It has been shown that 1% of circulating B lymphocytes in humans produce anti $\alpha_{1,3}$ Gal antibodies as a reaction to gastrointestinal bacteria. The first target for the genetic engineering at pigs as organ donors has been to knock out the pig gene for $\alpha_{1,3}$ GT. This was achieved through gene targeting and nuclear transfer (Cooper, 2003). In xenotransplantation another potential problem is porcine endogenous retrovirus (PERV) to the recipient. To reduce the release of PERV by porcine transplants, a new approach, using synthetic short interfering RNAs (siRNAs) corresponding to the different part of the viral genes gag, pol and env was applied by Karlas et al. (2004). This strategy was efficient in suppression of PERV replication.

Another group of animals with potential as organ donors is fish. A group of Canadian investigators has produced transgenic tilapia in which the islets of β cells in the Brockmann body synthesis human insulin. These transgenic fish could serve as donor of islets for xenotransplantation, even in the encapsulated from form (immuno-isolated), because they display higher hypoxia resistance than mammal (Pohajdak *et al.*, 2004). Advantages of this xenotransplantation is low cost and do not cause any zoonotic infection to recipient.

Application of as animal model for human disease

The animal model used for studying human disease process is the mice. Disease studied using the transgenic mouse model includes sickle cell anemia, amyotrophic lateral sclerosis, chronic hypertension, renal degeneration, osteogenesis imperfeita, cystic fibrosis, mitochondrial cardiomyopathy, neurodegenerative disease, Werner syndrome, rhodopsin mutation, retinitis pigmentosa, melanoma, Alzheimer's disease, prostate cancer and atherosclerosis (Venkateswaran *et al.*, 2004) mutamouse and big blue are transgenic mouse strains currently used for mutagenicity tensing (Mepham *et al.*, 1998).

Transgenic rabbits used as an animal model for human cardiovascular disease and atherosclerosis (Bosze *et al.*, 2003). The transgenic pigs used as large animal model for human eye disease retinitis pigmentosa (Petters *et al.*, 1997).

Current risks in Transgenesis

Cost of production

The operational cost of making transgenic mouse is about Rs. 4,400 making an expressing transgenic livestock founder can cost approximately anywhere between 11,00,000 and Rs. 2,20, 00,000 (Wall *et al.*, 1992).

Success rate

Still using different method of transgenesis, the success rate is less than 10% only due to multifactorial problem.

Animal health

Insertion of a transgene may upset the expression of the genome of host animal (and the consequence functioning of the animal)

Table : Current Company producing transgenic products

Species	Company	Website	Products	Status
Goats	GTC Biotherapeutics (USA)	http://www.transgenics.com	Antithrombin III, Monoclonal antibodies, Malaria vaccine	Completed European efficacy study (AT – III)
	Nexin Biotechnologies (Canada)	http://www.dexiabiotech.co	Spider silk Protein, Herman	Other products in preclinical Fiber development research
Cattle	Hematrech (USA)	http://www.hematech.com	Human polyclonal antibodies (vaccines)	Research
	GTC biotherapeutics (USA)	http://www.transgenics.com	Human serum albumin	Research
Sheep	PPL (UK)	http://www.ppl-therapeutics.com	Alpha 1 antitrypsin	Trials postponed Assets business being gold
Rabbit	Pharming (Netherlands)	http://www.pharming.com	C1 – inhibitor	Phase II clinical trials
	Bioprotein Technologies (France)	http://www.bioprotein.com	Recombinant protein	Research
Chicken	Vivalice (France)	http://www.vivalis.com		
	Avigenics. Inc (USA)	http://www.avigenics.com	Recombinant Proteins	Research
	Transxenogen (USA)	http://www.tranxenogen.com		
	Virage (USA)	http://www.virage.com		

Virus transfer

This is particular concern in animal bred as tissue donor for xenotransplantation, but now a day it can be over come with help of siRNAs, shRNA technique.

Dissemination

Normal reproduction may result in a transgene being released to the wild population.

Conclusion

Currently many companies start producing gene farming for therapeutic protein (listed in table 3) but now USA is the first country approved products were obtained in transgenic systems in last week of December 2006. Currently anti-thrombin III proteins produced in transgenic animals just completed the regulatory process. Many biopharmaceuticals proteins are under clinical trails and some are awaiting for regulatory approvement. We expect many transgenic therapeutic protein reaches the commercial market with in a decade. If it happens, it going to good revolution in transgenic animal production and pharmaceuticals industry and that will helpful in economic uplifting of poor farmers. Using modern technique such as knocking out siRNAs, shRNA and ribozymes along with transgenesis. We can remove particular receptor (that makes the animal susceptible to disease) and there by we can make disease resistant herd and other hand we can stamp out zoonotic disease to human beings.

References

Arezzo, F. Sea urchine sperm as a reactor of foreign genetic information.Cell.Biol. 1989; 13:391 – 394.

Bawden, C.S., Powell, B.C., Walker, S.K. and Roger, G.E. Expression of wool intermediate filament keratin transgene in sheep fiber alters structure. Transgenic Res. 1998; 7:273- 287.

Bleck, G.T., White, B.R., Miller, D.J. and Wheeler, M.B. production of bovine a- lactalbumin in the milk of transgenic pigs.J. Anim. Sci. 1998; 76: 3072-3078.

Bosze, Z.S., Hiripi, L., Carnwath, J.W. and Wiemann, H. the transgenic rabbit as model for human disease and as a source of biologically active recombinant proteins. Transgenic Res. 2003; 12:541-553.

Bowen, R.A., Reed, M., Schnieke, A., Seidal, G.E., Staacy, A., Thomas, W.K. and Kaijkawa, O. Transgenic cattle resulting from biopsies embryos expression of *c-ski* in a transgenic calf.Biology of reproduction.1994; 50: 664-668.

Bracket, B.G., Baranska, W., Sawichi, W. and Korpwski, H. Uptake of heterologous genome bymammalian spermatozoa and it transfer to ova through fertilization. Pro.Natl.Acade.Sci.1971; 68:353-357.

Brink, M.F., Bishop, M.D. and Pipeper, F.R. Developing efficient strategies for the generation of transgenic cattle which produce biopharmaceuticals in milk.Theriogenology.2000; 53:139-148.

Bueler, H., Aguzzi, A., Sailer, A., Groniner, R.A., Autonrined, P., Aguest, M. and Weissman, C. Mice devoid as PrP are resistant to scrapie.Cell.1993; 73:1339-1347.

Cen, L.R., Shiue, Y.L., Bortoline, L., Medrano, J.P., Bondurant, R.H. and Anderson,G.B. Establishment of pluripotent cell line from porcine Preimplantation embryos.Theriogenology.1999; 52:195-212.

Collores, T., Bongalhard, D.C., Deschamps, J.C. and Moreira, H.L.M. Transgenic animals: the melding of molecular biology and animal reproduction. Animal Reprod. 2005; 2(1): 1-27.

Cooper, D.K.C. Clinical xenotransplantation how close are we?.Lancet.2003; 362:557-559.

Dyck, M.K., Gangne, D., Quelled, M., Seneschal, J.F., Balanger, E., Larcroix, D., Strard, M.A. and Pother, F. Seminal vesicle production and secretion of growth hormone into seminal fluid. Nat.Biotechnol.1999; 17:1087-1090.

Golovan, S.P., Medinger, R.G., Sjakaiye, A., Cottrill, M., Wiedekehr, M.Z., Barnehy, D.J., Plante, C., Pollardj. W., Fan, M.N., Hayes, M.A., Laursen, J., Hiorth, J.P., Hacker, R.R., Philips,J.W.and Forsberg, C.W. Pig expressing salivary phytase produce low phosphorous manure. Nat. Biotechnol. 2001; 19:741-745.

Gordon, J.W and Ruddle, F.H. Integration and stable germ line transmission of genes inserted into mouse pronuclei. Science.1981; 214:1244-1246.

Gordon, J.W., Scangos, G.A., Poltkin, D.J., Barbosa, J.A. and Ruddle, F.H. Genetic transformation of mouse embryos by microinjection of purified DNA. Pro.Natl.Acad.Sci.USA. 1980; 77:7380-7384.

Grosvanor, C.E., Picciano, P. and Baumrucker, C.R. hormones and growth factors in milk.Endocriol. Rev. 1993; 14(6):710-728.

Haller, O., Arnheiter, H., Gresser, E. and Lindenmann, J. Virus specific interferon action/protection of newborn *Mx* carries against lethal infection with influenza virus. J. Exp.Med. 1981; 154:199-203.

Harris, J.W., Strong, D.D., Amoui, M., Baylink, D.J. and Lau, K.H. construction at a tcl- like transposon sleeping beauty based gene transfer plasmid vector for regeneration of stable transgenic mammalian cell clone. Analytic Biochemistry.2002; 310:15-26.

Houdebin, L.M. Transgenesis to improve animal production. Livestock Prod Sci. 2002; 74:255 – 268.

Hout, V.D. Long term intravenous treatment of pompe's disease with recombinant human 2 glucosidase from milk.Pediatric.2004; 113:448-457.

Imoto, T., Johnson, L.N., North, A.T., Philips, D.C. and Rupley, J.A. Vertebrate lysozyme. In:The enzyme vol.7 P.D. Boyer, (Ed), Academic Press, New York.NY. pp.665-868.

Ivics, Z., Hckett, P.B., Plasterk, R.H. and Izsvak, Z. Molecular reconstruction of sleeping beauty a *tcl* – like transposon from fish and its transposition in human cells. Cell.1997; 91:501-510.

Jaenisch, R., Pan, H. and Crocker, B. Infection of Preimplantation mouse embryos and of new born mice with leukemia virus: tissue distribution of viral DNA and RNA leukenogenesis in adult animal. Proc. Natl. Acade. Sci. USA.1975; 72:4008 – 4012.

Kawabe, X., Kamihira, M., Ono, I., Yogoku, K., Nishijima, K.I. and Iijima, S. Production of $SCF_v - F_c$ fusion protein using genetically manipulated quails. J. Bio Sci. Bio Eng. 2006; 102(4):297-303.

Keefer, C.L. Production of bioproducts through the use of transgenic animal models.Animal Reprod. Sci. 2004; 83:5-12.

Kerr, D.E., Liang, F., Bonodioli, K.R., Zhoo, H., Kreibich, G., Wall, R.J. and Sun, T.T.The bladder as a bioreactor, urothelium production and secretion at growth hormone into urine. Nat. Biotechnol.1998; 16:75-79.

Lavitrano, M., Frenc, D., Zani, M., Frati, L. and Syadatora, C.The interaction between exogenous DNA and sperm cells.Mole.Reprod.Dev. 1992; 31:161-169.

Lewin, H.A. Disease resistance and immuno response gene in cattle: strategies for their detection and evidence of their existence. J. Dairy Sci. 1989; 72:1334- 1348.

Limonta, J.M., Castro, F.O., Matinez, R., Puentes, P., Ramos, B., Aguilar, A., Lieonart, R.L. and Fuente, J.L. Transgenic rabbits as bioreactor for the production of human growth hormone. J. Biotechnol. 1995; 40:49-58.

Logan, J.S. Prospects for xenotransplantation.Curr.Opin.Immuno.2000; 12:563-568.

Mcpherron, A.C., Lawler, A.M. and Le, S.J. Regulation of skeletal muscle mass in mice by TGF- beta super family member.Nature.1997; 387: 83-90.

Mepham, T.B., Combes, R.D., Balls, M., Barbieri, O., Blokhuis, H.J., Costa, P., Crilly, R.E., Burninh, T.D.C., Delpire, V.C., Harge, M.J.O., Houdebine, L.M., Kroijl, C.F.V., Meer, M.V.D., Reinhardt, C.A., Wold, E. and Zeller, A.M.V. The use of transgenic animals in European Union.ATLA.1998; 26:21-43.

Muller, M., Brening, B., Winnacker, E.L., and Brem, G. Transgenic pigs carrying cDNA copies encoding the marine *Mxl* protein which confers resistance to influenza virus infection. Gene. 1992; 121(2):263- 270.

Oftedal, O.T. Milk composition, milk yield and energy output at peak lactation: a comparative review. In: physiological strategies in lactation. Peaker *et al.,* 1984. (Ed), Academic Press, London. PP. 33-86.

Onishi, A., Wamoto, M.I., Akita, T., Mikawa, S., Takeda, K., Awata, T., Hanada, H. and Perry, A.C.P. Pig cloning by microinjection of fetal fibroblast nuclei.Science.2000; 289:1180-1190.

Palmiter, R.D., Brinster, R.L., Hammer, R.E., Trumbauer, M.E., Rosenfeld, M.G., Birnberg, N.C. and Evans, R.M. Dramatic growth of mice that develop from eggs microinjected with metallothionein growth hormone fusion gene.Nature.1982; 300: 611-615.

Parry R.M. Transgenic livestock as genetic models of human disease. Reprod. Fert.Dev. 1994; 6:643-645.

Petters, R.M., Alexander, C.A., Nells, K.D.,Collin, E.B., Sommer, J.R., Blanton, M.R., Rajos, G., Hao, Y., Flowors, W.L., Banin, E., Cideciyan, A.V., Jacobson, S.C. and Wong, F. Genetically engineered large animal model for studying cone photoreceptor survival and degeneration in retinitis pigmentosa. Nat. Biotechnology. 1997; 15:965-970.

Pinkert, C. Transgenic animal biotechnology. Pinkert, C.A.: Academic Press.

Ponajdak, B., Mansour, O., Conlon, H.J.M., Dymond, L.C. and Wright, J.R. Production at transgenic tilapia with Brockmann bodies secreting human insulin. Transgenic Res. 2004; 13:313-323.

Pursel, V.G. Can you tell if any of these animals are transgenic? Your world biotechnonology and you. 1995; 5(1): 1- 16.

Rudolph, N.S. Biopharmaceutical production in transgenic livestock.Trends Biotechnol.1999; 17:376- 374.

Sachs, D.H., Sykes, M., Robson, S.C. and Cooper, K.C. Xenotransplantation. Adv. Immunol. 2001; 79:129-223.

Sato, M., Ishikawa, A., and Kimura,M. 2002. Direct injection of foreign DNA into mouse testis as a possible in vivo gene transfer system via epididymal spermatozoa.Mol. Reprod.Dev. 2002;61:45-49.

Sawanson, M.E., Martin, M.J., Donnell, J.K.O., Hoover, K., Lago, W., Huntress, V., Parson, C.T. and Pinkert, C.A. Production of functional haemoglobin in transgenic swine. Nat. Biotechnol. 1992; 10:557-559.

Scott, B.B. and Locks, C. Generation of transgenic birds with replication-deficient lenti viruses.Nature Protocol. 2006; 1(3): 1406-1411.

Setchell, B.P. In:The physiology of reproduction (ed). Knobile and Neil. J. Raven press Ltd. New york. 1988.pp. 753-836.

Spadafora, C. Sperm cells and foreign DNA: a controversial relation. Bioassays.1998; 20:955-964.

Sutrave, P., Kellys, A.M. and Hughes, S.H. *Ski* can cause selective growth at skeletal muscle in transgenic mice. Genes Dev. 1990; 4:1462 – 1472.

Thiemann, W.J. and Palladino, M.A. Introduction to biotechnology. In: Animal biotechnology. Ed. Benjamin comings, 1310 Sansome Street, San Francisco, CA 94111, pp. 153-168.

Tsunoday, Y. and Kato, Y. Nuclear transplantation of embryonic stem cells in mice. J. Reprod. Fertility.1993; 98:537-540.

Umadevi, S. 2006. Enzyme in poultry feeding recent development.Summer school on recent advance in the feed additive for production of residue free livestock/poultry products. pp. 64-68.

Vermus, H. Retroviruses. Science.1998; 240:1427-1435.

Venkateswaran, V., Flesner, N.E., Sugar, L.M. and Klotz, L.H. antioxidants block prostate cancer in lady transgenic mice. Cancer Res. 2004; 15:5891-5896.

Vise, P.P., Michalska, A.E., Ashuman, R., Lloyd, B., Stone, A.B., Quinn, P., Wells, J.R.E. and Seamark, R.R. Introduction of a porcine growth hormone fusion gene into transgenic pigs promoters growth. J. Cell. Sci. 1998; 90:295-300.

Wakayama, T.A., Perry, A.C.F., Zucott, M., Johnson, K.K. and Yanagimachi, R. Full term development of mice from enucleated oocyte injected with cumulus cell nuclei.Nature.1998; 394:369-374.

Wall, R.J. Biotechnology for the production of modified innovative animal product, transgenic livestock bioreactors. Livestock Production Science. 1999; 59:243-255.

Wall, R.J., Hawak, H.W. and Nel, N. Making transgenic livestock: genetic engineering on a large scale. J. Cell Biochem. 1992; 49:113-120.

Wall, R.J., Hyman, P., Kerr, D., Pintado, B. and Wells, K. Transgenic animal technology. J. Andrology. 1997; 18(3):236-239.

Whitelaw, C.B.A. Transgenic livestock made easy. TRENDS Biotechnol.2004; 22:157-159.

Whitelaw, C.B.A. and Sang, H.M. Disease resistant genetically modified animals. Rev. Sci. Tech. Off. Int. Epiz. 2005; 24(1):275-283.

Wilmut, I. and Paterson, L. Somatic cell nuclear transfer.Oncology Research.2003; 13:303-307.

❑❑❑

Chapter 4

Micro and Nano-Scale Technologies : Applications in Bovine Reproduction Research

GOKULDAS P.P * AND PERUMAL P **
*Scientist (Animal Reproduction), NRC on Pig, Guwahati, Assam
**Scientist (Animal Reproduction), NRC on Mithun, Nagaland

Miniature technologies, especially at molecular and nanoscale level, are progressing rapidly during the past two decades. So called nanotechnology is now considered as one of the most prominent actors of scientific revolution marking the new millennium. The science of nanotechnology have the ability to work at the atomic, molecular and even sub-molecular levels in order to create and use material structures, devices and systems with new properties and functions. It is extremely diverse and multidisciplinary field, ranging from novel extensions of conventional device physics, to completely new approaches based upon molecular self-assembly to developing new materials with dimensions on the nanoscale. The progress made by the nanotechnology in different scientific fields has been astonishing with many of the western countries planning mammoth funding for this research. Microfluidics is another promising area which makes use of technology that not only sorts sperm and eggs but also brings them together in a way that mimics the movement of natural reproduction and then handles the resulting embryo. Such a technique would make mass production of embryos cheap, quick and reliable.

Even though, application of nanotechnology and other miniature technologies in animal reproduction is still in infancy, it is predicted to revolutionize livestock sector with countless ground breaking innovations. This chapter is a humble effort to highlight the significance and future prospects of nanotechnology with special emphasis on its applications in bovine reproduction.

What is Nanotechnology?

Nanotechnology is the engineering of functional systems at the molecular or nano-scale level. It is a research and development aimed at understanding and working with seeing, measuring and manipulating matter at the atomic, molecular and supramolecular levels.

This correlates to length scales of roughly 1 to 100 nanometres. Nanotechnology has been defined by the U.S. National Nanotechnology Initiative (NNI) as "understanding and control of mater at dimensions of roughly 1 to 100nm where unique phenomena enable novel applications".

At this scale, the physical, chemical and biological properties of materials differ fundamentally and often unexpectedly. Through these unique properties, nanotechnology can provide new tools for molecular and cellular biology, biotechnology, veterinary physiology, reproduction and many more. Now even converging technologies are shaped resulting from merger of nanotechnology with biomedicine, bio-sciences, biotechnology and genetic engineering. Nanobiotechnology is defined as a field that applies the nanoscale principles and techniques to understand and transform biosystems (living or non-living) and which uses biological principles and materials to create new devices and systems integrated from the nanoscale.

Nanomaterials

Nanomaterials are structures created by nanotechnology research that range from 1 to 100 nanometers in size. Common examples of nanomaterials found in scientific literature are *nanotubes, fullerenes, quatumdots, dendrimers,buckyballs* and *nanoshells*. Nanomaterials can have very different properties than materials at the macro scale. They can be stronger, lighter, more electrically conductive, more porous and less corrosive than bulk materials.

Nanotubes are a sequence of nanoscale C-60 atoms arranged in a long thin cylindrical structure. **Fullerenes** are pure carbon molecules composed of at least 60 atoms of carbon. By definition, **Quantum dots** are a nano-scale crystalline structure made from cadmium selenide that absorbs white light and then reemits it a couple of nanoseconds later in a specific color. **Dendrimers** are synthetic, technically a polymer, three-dimensional macromolecules formed using a nanoscale fabrication process. **Nanoshells** are concentric sphere nanoparticles consisting of a dielectric (typically gold sulfide or silica) core and a metal (gold) shell. They are considered a very special kind of nanoparticle because they combine infrared optical activity with the uniquely biocompatible properties of gold colloid.

How miniature technologies are set to impact bovine reproduction?

Nanotechnology and related miniature technologies have the potential to solve many more puzzles related to animal health, reproduction, production, good hygienic practices during rearing and maintaining of food animals. Although much research and major company developments are necessary before nanotechnology is common place in veterinary and animal sciences, there are numerous glimpses of applications as discussed below.

Accurate estrus detection

Management of breeding is an expensive and time-consuming problem for dairy and swine farmers. It is now possible to accurately monitor animal hormone levels using an implantable nano-sensing device with wireless transmission capability. In this way the information of optimal fertility period would be available in real time to assist the livestock operators. One solution that is currently being studied is a nanotube implanted under the skin to provide real time measurement of changes in the level of estradiol in the blood. The nanotubes (O'Connell *et al.*, 2002) are used as a means of tracking oestrus in animals because these tubes have the capacity to bind and detect the estradiol antibody at the time of oestrus by near infrared fluorescence. The signal from this sensor will be incorporated as a part of a central monitoring and control system to actuate breeding. It is an interesting area in reproductive management which can be exploited for prompt heat detection, ovulation time and pregnancy diagnosis.

Artificial Insemination and semen cryopreservation

Nanoscale delivery systems can significantly improve bioavailability and better control of release kinetics, reduce labour intensity, and minimize waste and discharge to the environment. Researchers in Brazil are working on Fixed-Time Artificial Insemination (FTAI) technology combined with nanotechnologies to effectively increase the success rate in cattle reproduction.FTAI depends on the regulation of progesterone administered through a silicone matrix.Development of novel applications of nanostructured silica in medicine, biotechnology and reproduction, has been primary focus at various nanotechnology institutes. Fumed silica, when included in cell suspensions, demonstrates high adhesion to the cell surface. Chemical and adsorption modification of the surface of nanoparticles by biologically active molecules diversify the spectrum of possible effects of nanostructured silica. Nanosize fumed silica, used as a carrier in proposed nanomaterials, has been proved to provide itself the positive biological effect with respect to reproductive cells especially sperms. New silica based nanomaterials as admixtures to existing cryomedia were synthesized and successfully tested with post thaw bovine sperm to increase their viability and longevity.

Enhancing semen quality

Many studies have shown that Selenium is required for the maintenance of bull fertility. Recently, nano-elemental selenium has attracted wide spread attention due to its high bioavailability and low toxicity because nanometer particulates exhibit novel characteristics, such as great specific surface area, high surface activity, a lot of surface active centers, high catalytic efficiency and strong adsorbing ability and the character of low toxicity of routine Selenium. Supplementation with nano-Se has been found to enhance testicular Selenium content, testicular and semen GSH-Px activity, and protect the membrane system integrity and the tight arrangement of the midpiece of the mitochondria.

Transgenic animal production

Genetic engineering of livestock is faced with technical challenges that nanotechnology might be able to overcome. In this category, two examples of genetic engineering through the use of nanoparticles are currently under investigation. The first uses nanoparticles bound on a matrix to deliver DNA into bovine embryos for temporal expression and selection of genes. The second involves free-standing nanoparticles to deliver genes into embryos for germline modification of livestock or into adult animal tissues for gene therapy. A novel method of DNA delivery has recently been described using arrays of vertically aligned carbon nanofibers (VACNFs). Cells are pressed onto the DNA-coated VACNFs which then penetrate the cells and introduce the DNA. They could help to overcome the tedious microinjection involved in genetic manipulation of livestock as well as allow for the temporal expression of genes that are not introduced into the inheritable genetic material of embryos but could affect them at crucial times.

Improving nutritional status

A critical element for sustainable bovine reproduction is the improvement of nutritional status of the animal. Nanotechnologies may offer significant improvements here as well. As with food applications, a variety of nanoscale delivery systems have been investigated in feeds to facilitate utilization of proteins and improve the overall health of animals to maintain optimal physiological and reproductive state. In addition, nanoscale delivery systems can be designed for veterinary drug delivery, which protects the drug through the gastro-intestinal tract and allows the release at the desired location for best effect. These advantages improve the efficiency by which animals utilize nutrient resources, help reduce the material and financial burden of the producers, and improve product quality and production yield.

Molecular Imaging (nanobioimaging)

The use of nanoparticles for imaging has gained considerable momentum in recent years. Fluorescent Quantum Dots (QDs), which are small nanocrystals (1–10 nm) made of inorganic semiconductor materials, possess several unique optical properties best suited for in vivo imaging. In addition, QDs are extremely photostable, making them ideally suited for long-term observations or repeated measurements. Atomic force microscopy (AFM) has emerged as the only technique capable of real-time imaging of the surface of a living cell at nano-resolution. AFM provides the advantage of directly observing living biological cells in their native environment and thus proved to be a valuable tool for reproductive biologists. The ability of this technique to image non-conductive living cells in physiological environment (aqueous solution) in 3D array without elaborate sample preparation or fixing of samples unlike conventional electron microscopy (which requires the cells to be fixed with aldehyde and stained) has made AFM a valuable tool to study various biomolecules, including sperm cells. Unstained, unfixed bovinr spermatozoa in their natural physiological surroundings can be imaged by this technique which provides valuable information about the morphological and pathological defects in sperm cells as thrée-dimensional images with precise topographical details. Sperm head defects and the acrosome at the tip of the head responsible for fertilization, can be examined and correlated with the lack of functional integrity of the cell.

Microfluidics: "Lab-on-a-chip" technology

Microfluidics is now an established miniature technology that shows promise as an alternative in the process of embryo in vitro production (IVEP). It is a technology that allows a fresh examination of the way assisted reproduction is performed. It is based on the behaviour of liquids in a microenvironment. Although a young field, many developments have occurred which demonstrate the potential of this technology for gamete and embryo manipulation.

Microfluidic devices vary greatly in design and are used in a variety of scientific disciplines, including Assisted Reproductive Technologies.

Studies have shown advantages of media flow in microfluidic devices for all aspects of ART, including sperm processing in-*vitro* maturation, fertilization and embryo culture. With the development of nano-devices, scientists are able to investigate cells at the single cell, cellular, and sub-cellular levels using methods that were not available a few years ago. The development of ef?cient, reliable culture systems for single embryos or gametes (sperm or oocytes) will provide new avenues to study the microenvironment experienced by these unique cells. The microchannel culture systems using microfluidic technology provide an embryo culture environment that more closely mimics the *in vivo* environment and help in faster embryonic development.

Microfluidic technology uses minimal amounts of media in a constricted environment, similar to that experienced by gametes and embryos *in vivo*. This "lab-on-a-chip" would not only save space, but also time, as it allows for automation of processes as well as inclusion of diagnostic assays aimed at non-invasively identifying the healthiest cells for subsequent use. Interestingly, methods designed to separate motile sperm using micro?uidic devices have been reported which uses a nanotechnique in which tiny laser tractor beams trap individual sperm and then sort them by weight. This technique can sort around 3,000 sperm per second, and aims for commercialisation in cattle breeding. Microfluidics remains one of the most exciting modern scientific developments and continues to have a tremendous impact on embryo biotechnology and in vitro embryo production.

Cell micro-encapsulation

Cell encapsulation is an evolving branch of biotechnology with numerous applications including the enhancing of reproductive performance both in humans and farm animals. It is a strategy whereby a pool of live cells is entrapped within a semipermeable membrane. Over the last twenty years male and female gametes and embryos have been encapsulated with or without somatic cells, for different purposes, such as semen controlled release, in vitro gametogenesis, embryo culture after in vitro fertilization and cell preservation.

The first application of cell encapsulation in mammal reproduction was made by Nebel and coworkers who devised a technique for bovine sperm encapsulation in calcium alginate and polyamines. They introduced the idea of spermatozoa controlled release and the targeting of the female reproductive system for artificial insemination: high sperm concentrations can be maintained in the bovine uterus during the ovulation, thus, guaranteeing an increase in fertility and prolificacy. Since then, the applications of cell microencapsulation in reproductive biotechnologies have been expanded to other fields with different aims. Researches have obtained satisfactory in vivo fertilization results in CIDR synchronized heifers. They observed an increase in fertility with encapsulated semen at the optimal time of insemination (48 hours after CIDR removal). As well as gamete preservation, valid micro-encapsulation methods have been established for the amelioration of in vitro conditions for the preservation and the early development of in vitro-obtained bovine embryos and thus to improve IVF yield.

Use of biosensors

A biosensor is an analytical device, consisting of bio-recognition system (typically enzymes or antibodies) that is either closely connected to, or integrated within, a physico-chemical transducer (electrochemical, optical, piezoelectric or thermometric). The biosensor responds to the presence of a specific analyte by producing an electric signal that is proportional to the concentration of the analyte. The bio-receptor selectivity provides the opportunity for the development of highly specific devices for real-time analysis in complex mixtures, without the need for sample pre-treatment. Biosensors also promise to be highly sensitive, rapid, reproducible and simple-to-operate analytical tools.

Nanotechnology is playing an increasingly important role in the development of biosensors and various nanoparticles have emerged as powerful and widely applicable materials in biosensing. By conjugating specific molecules to the surface of nanoparticles, it is possible to engineer their biological functionality. An exciting product of the progress in nanoparticles for in vitro diagnostic tools has been the emergence of probes encapsulated by biologically localized embedding (PEBBLEs).

They are nanoscale polymer beads specifically designed to provide minimally invasive monitoring of specific analytes in single, viable cells with applications for real-time analysis of drugs, toxins, and environmental effects on cell function. Another group of nanoparticles for biosensing are quantum dots (QDs). When excited with a beam of photons, they emit bright light at a distinct frequency on their own and hence are a promising technology for many biosensing applications especially in the field of *in vivo* imaging.

For several years progesterone in milk or blood has been recognized as an indicator of different cow states related to reproduction. If cow level information on progesterone level is available as a routine, and especially, if automated, it might be possible to improve reproductive efficiency. With the advent of biosensors, attempts at automation and inline application of quantitative enzyme immunoassays for progesterone have been reported. Recently, development of a novel progesterone biosensor system which can sample milk from the line on demand by the computer and pulled it to a central point where it can be analysed with a disposable biosensor, have been reported. Scientists are also trying to develop a fully automated ovulation prediction system for dairy cows. The device operates in a competitive immunoassay format and relies on a reduction in the binding of alkaline phosphatase-labelled progesterone to the sensor surface in the presence of endogenous milk progesterone. The results from field-tests show that the progesterone biosensor can characterize the ovulation cycles of cows and detect pregnancy.

Future prospects of the technology

Fertility Chip

A new 'fertility chip', developed by researchers at the University of Twente's MESA+ Institute for Nanotechnology, can accurately count spermatozoa in sperm. This is an important step towards the development of a compact device for reliable 'pre-scanning' of male fertility. The chip has the ability to accurately count spermatozoa. On the new chip, the spermatozoa flow through a fluid channel, above which electrodes are fitted. When a cell flows under this 'bridge', its electrical resistance changes momentarily, and this event is counted. There is nothing wrong to hope that one day this technology could be effectively expoited in animal sector. Further research will need to establish whether quality characteristics can be measured in a similar manner, so that a compact device can be developed in which chip can be inserted for single use.

Prenatal diagnostics

Ultrasound and other monitoring technologies have transformed the way prenatal and neonatal care is provided as well as the process of parturition. Other emerging trends in animal monitoring are likely to be the integration of nanotechnology and state-of-the-art technologies such as bio micro-electromechanical systems (bio MEMS) micro-processors. These innovative micro- and nanosensing devices are likely to be monitoring aids in the future with applications in fetal pulse monitoring and pulse oximetry.

Nano-ultrasonography

Detailed information on 3D topographical images of spermatozoa acquired by AFM is expected to provide a better understanding of various reproductive pathways which, in turn, can facilitate improved infertility management and/or contraceptive development. The shape of gamete, zygote, embryo and foetal development at nano-level shall bring forth new additions to our knowledge. Combing cognitive, mythical and mysterious happening within the uterus could be registered and translated via nano-ultrasonography.

Nano-electronic technologies

Many nanotechnology companies are currently performing early-stage research for the development of novel hormone sensor/meter for biomedical applications in the areas of infertility in humans. Companies have licensed carbon nanotube technology which increases hormonal detection sensitivity significantly, allowing detection beyond traditional biosensors. The company is using this technology to develop biomedical applications that are low in power consumption and small in size and that involve ultra-sensitive nanoelectronic technologies.

In the future, nanoparticles that are engineered with specific binding affinities towards reproductive hormones can be resuspended into the collected body fluids, or perhaps even injected directly into the circulation. The nanoparticles, together with the bound molecules, could be directly captured on engineered filters and directly questioned by ultra high-resolution mass spectrometry. New micro-encapsulation technologies are going to be patented over the coming years: these will include standardized procedures for large scale capsule production for bovine artificial insemination as well as easy-to-use kits for "homemade" capsules, which could be routinely used in the therapy of human reproductive disorders.

Conclusion

Nanotechnology will leave no field untouched by its ground breaking scientific innovations. It can provide new tools for molecular and cellular biology, biotechnology, reproduction, veterinary physiology and animal genetics. The applications of nanotechnology to animal production are very diverse. Nanotechnology has a tremendous potential to revolutionize agriculture and livestock sector. Nanotechnology tools like microfluidics, nanomaterials, bioanalytical nanosensors, etc. have the potential to solve many more puzzles related to animal reproduction, production and health. The continued progress in the development and use of micro- and nanotechnologies shows great potential in improving methods to diagnose diseases or to monitor reproductive status of animals. So far, the use of nanotechnology in the animal sector has been mostly theoretical, but it has begun and will continue to have a significant effect in the main areas of the medicine and reproduction.

References

Aneeve Nanotechnologies to Develop Sensors to Monitor Hormone Levels for Menopause and Fertility.Available online at http://www.azonano.com/news.asp?newsID=15367

Cabrera, L., Heo, Y., Ding, J. and Smith, G. (2006). Improved blastocyst development with microfluidics and braille pin actuator enabled dynamic culture. *Fertil Steril*; **87**: S43.

Chaudhry, Q., Scotter, M., Blackburn, J., Ross, B., Boxall, A., Castle, L., Aitken, R. and Watkins, R. 2008.Applications and implications of nanotechnologies for the food sector. Food Addit Contam 25 (3): 241-58.

Claycomb, R.W. and Delwiche, M.J. (1998).Biosensor for on-line measurement of bovine progesterone during milking. Biosens Bioelectron. 15;13(11):1173-80.

Convenient biochip to allow accurate semen analysis at home. Available online at http://www.chinapost.com.tw/health/sexual-health-/2009/09/16/224936/Convenient-biochip.htm

Feneque, J. (2003). Brief introduction to the veterinary applications of nanotechnology.Nano-technology now. Website: www.nanotech-now.com/Jose-Feneque/Veterinary Appliations-Nanotechnology.htm

Feneque, J.: Nanotechnology: a new challenge for veterinary medicine. The Pet Tribune. 6 (5): 16. 2000.

'Fertility chip' to accurately count spermatozoa in sperm.Available online at http://www.news-medical.net/news/20100216/Fertility-chip-to-accurately-count-spermatozoa-in-sperm.aspxAccessed on 27th May, 2010.

Feynman, R. 1961. There's plenty of room at the bottom: An invitation to enter a new field of Physics. In H.D. Gilbert (Ed), Miniaturization.New York Reinhold.

Gillis EH, Gosling JP, Sreenan JM, Kane M. (2002).Development and validation of a biosensor-based immunoassay for progesterone in bovine milk. J Immunol Meth;267:131–8.

Glasgow, I., H. Zeringue, D. Beebe, S. Choi, J. Lyman and M. Wheeler (2000) Individual embryo transport and retention on a chip, microTAS, 199-202.

Jha, R.K., Jha, P.K. and Guha, S.K. (2009). Smart RISUG: A potential new contraceptive and its magnetic fi eld-mediated sperm interaction. International Journal of Nanomedicine. 4:55.

Kricka, L., O. Heyner, W. Garside and P. Wilding (1993) Applications of a microfabricated device for evaluating sperm function, Clinical Chemistry, 39, 1944- 1947.

Maria N. Velasco-Garcia and Toby Mottram. (2001). Biosensors in the livestock industry: an automated ovulation prediction system for dairy cows. Trends in Biotechnology, 19:11.

McKnight, T.E., Melechko, A.V., Griffin, G.D., Guillorn, M.A., *et al.,* 2003. Intracellular integration of synthetic nanostructures with viable cells for controlled biochemical manipulation. Nanotechnology 14, 551–556.

Nanotechnologies in agriculture: new tools for sustainable development. In International Conference on Food and Agriculture Applications of Nanotechnologies.NANOAGRI 2010 June 20-25 2010 - Sao Pedro, SP, Brazil.

Nebel RL, Bame JH, Saacke RG, Lim F. Microencapsulation of bovine spermatozoa. J Anim Sci 1985; 60(6):1631-1639.

NSTC, (2004): Available online at www.nano.gov/html/res/fy04-pdf/fy04main.html.

O'Connell, M.J., *et al.* (2002): *Science,* 297: 593-596.

Pemberton RM, Hart JP, Mottram TT. (2001). An electrochemical immunosensor for milk progesterone using a continuous flow system. Biosens Bioelectron ;16:715–23.

Quantum Dots for In Vivo Small-Animal Imaging Laurent A. Bentolila, Yuval Ebenstein, and Shimon Weiss. J Nucl Med 2009; 50:493–496.

Scott, N., Chen, H., 2003. Nanoscale science and engineering for agriculture and food systems. A National Planning Workshop. November 18–19, 2002.

Segerink, L., Sprenkels, A., Braak, P., Vermes, I. and Berg, A. (2010).On-chip determination of spermatozoa concentration using electrical impedance measurements. *Lab on a Chip,* 10:397.

Seo D, Agca Y, Feng ZC, Critser JK. (2007). Development of sorting, aligning, and orienting motile sperm using micro?uidic device operated by hydrostatic pressure.*Micro?uid Nano?uid,*10:10.

Shibata, D., Ando, H., Iwase, A., Harata, T., Kikkawa, F. and Naruse, K. (2007). Analysis of sperm motility and fertilization rates after the separation by microfluidic sperm sorter made of quartz. *Fertil.Steril.***88**: S110.

Sunil Kumar, Koel Chaudhury, Prasenjit Sen and Sujoy K Guha. (2005). Atomic force microscopy: a powerful tool for high-resolution imaging of spermatozoa. *Journal of Nanobiotechnology* 2005, **3**:9.

Zhang, X., Chen, J., Sun, H. and Xu, C. (2009). Follicle-Stimulating Hormone Peptide Can Facilitate Paclitaxel Nanoparticles to Target Ovarian Carcinoma *In vivo. Cancer Research* 69, 6506.

Zhihong, M., Xiaohuia, L. and Weiling, F. (1999). A new sandwich-type assay of estrogen using piezoelectric biosensor immobilized with estrogen response element. *Anal. Commun.*,36, 281–283.

□□□

Chapter 5

Lifeline of Genetically Modified Crops for Livestock

TILLING TAYO
SMS, KVK, Arunachal Pradesh

Genetically modified plants are plants whose DNA is modified using genetic engineering techniques. In most cases the aim is to introduce a new trait to the plant which does not occur naturally in this species. Examples include resistance to certain pests, diseases or environmental conditions, or the production of a certain nutrient or pharmaceutical agent. Agriculture and livestock being the main stay of developing countries, the demand for livestock products increases dramatically as population increases. Moreover, with increasing urbanization and rising income in many parts of the developing world, per capita consumption of meat, milk, and eggs is expected to rise by about 2% (Delgado *et al.,* 1999). Global demand for meat is also forecast to increase more than 55% of current consumption by 2020, with most of the increase occurring in developing countries (Rosegrant *et al.,* 2001).

Thus the demand for feed grain will increase by 3% per year in developing countries and 0.5% in developed countries. On the average, less than 3 kg of feed grain are required to produce a kilo of livestock meat and less than a kilo of feed grain per kg of milk.

GM crops have indirectly benefited the livestock sector as they have increased yields of feed ingredient, have better quality traits, and are safer for livestock. As a source of livestock feed components, the relevant GM crops include corn, canola, cottonseed, and soybean. These crops are principally used in livestock feed rations either as an energy and/or protein source.

Needs for the developments of GM crops

a) Quality improvement

The convectional crops products, like rapeseed mustard oil cake (RMC), can be readily used as a protein supplement in ruminant's diets due to its availability and being cheaper than other oil cakes, having a high crude protein ranging from 34 to 38% (Bell, 1984), with a good balance of essential amino acid (Singhal, 1986). However, due to presence of anti-nutritional factor, erucic acid (43-57%) and high level of glucosinolates (150-240μmole/g) in seed meal (TERI, 2003), limits its potential use as a protein supplement in ruminants. Glucosinolates present in RMC following hydrolysis by endogenous enzyme, myrosinase yield a metabolite such as thiocyanate, isothiocyanate, oxazolidone-2-thiones and nitrile compounds. These metabolites are responsible for pungent smell and bitter taste of the compound feed, which adversely affect the palatability of the diet, reduce feed intake and increase milk thiocyanate thereby reducing the iodide content of milk (G.H Palin *et al.,* 2007), presence of goitrogens in milk from cows fed RMC may be of toxicological concern (Iwarrson and Nilson 1973; Papas *et al.,* 1979). This leads to the development of single or double low (00/ canola) varieties of rapeseed crops by plant breeders. Canada was first to developed canola verities. In recent years, significant efforts have been made by National Research Centre on Rapeseed-Mustard and All India Research Coordinated Project towards generation of (canola) low erucic acid and low glucosinolates strains of *B. juncea* and *B. napus* (Agnihotri and Kaushik, 1998).

Modified oil content and composition (e.g. polyunsaturated fatty acids such as linoleic acid, laureic acid) for maize, soybeans, rapeseed and other oil crops: These modified crops could be important in the fight against cardiovascular disease, obesity, and certain forms of cancer.

Golden rice – enrichment with carotenoids (provitamin A): This project produced a rice cultivar with enhanced levels of beta-carotene and other carotenoids, which are metabolic precursors of vitamin A. Because rice naturally contains only a negligible amount of beta-carotene, vitamin A deficiency is widespread in regions of the world where rice is a staple food.

Higher content of protein or amino acids, or modified amino acid composition for enhanced nutritional value: For example, LY038, a maize line with enhanced lysine content for improved animal feed quality. It is now awaiting authorisation in the EU.

b) Pestresistance

Bacillus thuringiensis, or Bt, is a bacterium that has attracted much attention for its use in pest control. The soil bacterium produces a protein that is toxic to various herbivorous insects. The protein, known as Bt toxin is produced in an inactive, crystalline form. When consumed by insects, the protein is converted to its active, toxic form (delta endotoxin), which in turn destroys the gut of the insect (Zhang and Feng, 2000). Bt preparations are commonly used in organic agriculture to control insects, as Bt toxin occurs naturally and is completely safe for humans. More than 100 different variations of Bt toxin have been identified in diverse strains of *Bacillus thuringiensis*. The different variations have different target insect specificity, for example, the toxins classified under Cry1a group target Lepidoptera (butterflies), while toxins in the Cry3 group are effective against beetles.

Researchers have used genetic engineering to take the bacterial genes needed to produce Bt toxins and introduce them into plants. If plants produce Bt toxin on their own, they can defend themselves against specific types of insects. This means farmers no longer have to use chemical insecticides to control certain insect problems. Biotechnology has opened up new avenues for natural protection for plants by providing new biopesticides, such as microorganisms, that are toxic to targeted crop pests but do not harm humans, animals, fish, birds or beneficial insects.

The first GM crop approved for cultivation in India is the "Bt-cotton" which confers resistance to boll worm which is a menace in cotton crop.

c) Disease resistance

Plants are susceptible to viral, bacterial and fungal diseases. Much progress has been made in evolving transgenic plants resistant to Fungi are responsible for a range of serious plant diseases such as blight, grey mould, bunts, powdery mildew, and downy mildew. Crops of all kinds often suffer heavy losses. Fungal plant diseases are usually managed with applications of chemical fungicides or heavy metals. In some cases, conventional breeding has provided fungus resistant cultivars. Besides combating yield losses, preventing fungal infection keeps crops free of toxic compounds produced by some pathogenic fungi. These compounds, often referred to as mycotoxins, can affect the immune system and disrupt hormone balances. Some species of *Fusarium* fungi produce fumonisin, a dangerous toxin that can kill horses and pigs and cause esophageal cancer in humans. Eliminating the corn borer from corn reduces growth of the fungi from the corn plant (Munkvold *et al.,* 1997, 1999) and increases the quality and yield of corn. Because the Bt proteins produced in the genetically enhanced corn plant serve as insecticides, they kill the corn borers before they do much damage to the corn plant, and the opportunity for fungal growth is decreased.

d) Herbicide resistant

Several crops have been genetically modified to be resistant to non-selective herbicides. Glyphosate-tolerant crop varieties have been developed and commercialized for corn, soybeans, canola, and cotton (Sidhu *et al.,* 2000). These transgenic crops contain genes that enable them to degrade the active ingredient in an herbicide, rendering it harmless. Farmers can thereby easily control weeds during the entire growing season and have more flexibility in choosing times for spraying. Herbicide resistant crops also facilitate low or no tillage cultural practices, which many consider to be more sustainable. Another advantage is that farmers can manage weeds without turning to some of the more environmentally suspect types of herbicides. Critics claim that in some cases, the use of herbicide resistant crops can lead to an increase in herbicide use, promote the development of herbicide resistant weeds, and damage biodiversity on the farm. Extensive ecological impact assessments have been addressing these issues. In comparison with conventional cropping systems, weed and animal populations were negatively affected by herbicide tolerant sugar beet and rapeseed, but biodiversity was increased with the use of herbicide tolerant maize. Currently, two herbicide resistant cropping systems are common for soybean, maize, rapeseed, and cotton: *RoundupReady* (active agent: glyphosate) and *Liberty Link* (active agent: glufosinate).

Approximately 90 million hectares or about 1.2 billion acres of genetically modified (GM) crops are currently grown worldwide. The main GM crops grown commercially are soybean (54.4 mha), corn (21.2 mha), cotton (9.8 mha), and canola (4.6 mha).

The introduction of GM crops has produced significant benefits to both farmers and consumers. GM crops have minimized the use of pesticides and provided higher crop yields; consumers benefited in the form of improved quality products (e.g., canola and soybean with modified oils). Currently, more than 80 GM crop events/lines have been approved for food and/or feed use.

Increased production of food and feed has to be generated from increased yield because there is limited opportunity to increase cultivated land area without adverse environmental impacts. Keeping these views in fact scientist and plants breeders started to develop an improved varieties of crops (genetically modified crops) to sustain the life of human as well as livestock's within a limited cultivated land. The present review provides an overview of potential use and safety assessments of GM crops in livestock feeding.

Development of GM Crop/Transgenic

The steps and process involve in the generation of GM crops or transgenic crops up to the introduction into the market.

- Make copies of the gene
- Transfer to plant tissue

- Regenerate plants
- Lab analysis and safety testing
- Development of a variety
- Field tests
- Approval by Government agencies
- Commercialization
- Monitoring of efficacy and safety

GM crops (%) as Feed Ingredients in Livestock Diets

Feed grain usage as a percentage of total crop production ranges from 18% for wheat, 52% for sorghum, 70% for corn, 75% for oats, to more than 90% of oil seed meals (Gilbert, 2000). Livestock producers in many parts of the world prefer corn grain and soybean meal for energy and/or protein source in both monogastric and ruminant diets.

About 90 million metric tons of GM corn grains are produced worldwide. Given that 70% of total corn grain production are used for livestock feed, then at least 65 million metric tons of GM corn grains are used in livestock diets annually. In the case of soybean, about 70 million metric tons of soybean meals derived from GM soybean are fed to livestock per annum (Phipps, 2002).

Organism used in GM crops

Transgenic crops currently approved for use as animal feed are modified for herbicide tolerance, insect resistance, modified oil content, and virus resistance. Many of the proteins expressed in GM crops have a history of safe usage and/or are similar to naturally occurring proteins. For example, insect resistant transgenic crops express proteins from *Bacillus thuringiensis* (Bt), a common soil-borne bacterium that has been commercially used worldwide as a microbial insecticide by organic farmers. Expressed proteins (CP4 EPSPS) in glyphosate herbicide tolerant GM crops are similar to endogenous EPSPS already present in foods (MacKenzie and McLean, 2002).

Biochemical Safety Assessment of GM Products

Extensive testing and a long approval process accompany every GM crop introduction. The approval process includes comprehensive analyses to ensure food, feed, and environmental safety before entering the marketplace.

In 1993 OECD formulated the concept of Substantial Equivalence as a starting point for the safety assessment of GM crops. The concept has since been developed further (OECD, 1996 and 1998) and has obtained broad international consensus and is applicable to both foods and feeds (Kuiper, *et al.,* 2001, Chesson, 2000).

The concept is based on the idea that existing crops can serve as the basis for comparing the properties of a GM crop with an appropriate counterpart considered safe as shown by a long history of safe use. Application of the concept is not a safety assessment per se but helps to identify similarities and differences between conventional and GM crops. Differences are then the subject of further investigation.

Agronomic, phenotypic and compositional analysis of key nutritional components is the basis for establishing substantial equivalence. Padgette *et al.,* (1996), and Taylor *et al.,* (1999), provide excellent examples of the compositional analyses conducted during this process. From the numerous reports in the published literature Table 2 illustrates some of the data which demonstrates that conventional and Roundup Ready soybean have similar composition as measured by laboratory analyses (Linderman *et al.,* 2002).

Table 1 : Compositional equivalence

	Soybean Meal	
Composition (% DM)	**Conventional varieties**	**Roundup Ready GM**
DM	90.3	91.0
Crude Protein	51.5	51.2
Neutral Detergent fibre	4.95	4.85
Lysine	3.16	3.09
Meth + Cystine	1.47	1.51

Safety assessment of GM Feeds in livestock's

Dairy Cows

Many feeding trials have been conducted to examine the safety and efficacy of GM feeds in both monogastric and ruminant livestock there was no any significant difference in terms of diet digestibility, feed intake, milk production milk composition, feed efficiency and live-weight gain of animals fed either GM or conventional feed ingredients (Clark and Ipharraguere, 2001). These studies clearly established that GM feed ingredients were nutritionally equivalent to their isogenic non-GM counterpart and to commercially available varieties and have been reviewed by Artim *et al.,* (2002). According to Singhal *et al.,* (2008), there were no any statistical significant variations in milk composition in terms of fat, protein, lactose, SNF and total solids content in dairy cows receiving Non Bt groups and Bt group. Milk composition of crossbred cows was found similar to that reported by Singhal *et al.* (2006). Presence of Bt protein (Cry1Ac) was not detected in the milk samples, collected at various intervals after incorporation of Bt cottonseed in the ration of cows. These observations were similar to those reported by Singhal *et al.,* (2001) while feeding Bt cottonseed, Castillo *et al.* (2001) while feeding BG II cottonseed and Folmer *et al.* (2002) on feeding Bt corn silage to lactating cows. Cry 1Ac protein was also not detected in the blood plasma samples, drawn at the end of experimental feeding period. These results suggest that the Cry1Ac protein consumed by cows through Bt cottonseed either got degraded in the rumen or not absorbed across the intestinal mucosa in to the blood circulation and the absence of Cry 1 Ac in the milk was obvious.

According to recent reviewed by Faust (2000) and Flachowsky and Aulrich (2001), transgenic DNA has not been found in milk, meat or eggs derived from animals receiving GM feed ingredients in their diets. Similarly no GM DNA could be detected in any of the milk samples tested. The detection limit for the test was established at 7.5 ug/l of milk. When DNA was extracted from the diet, the yield obtained was equivalent to 0.16 g 20 kg DM which was the average daily feed intake cow day at CEDAR and even if fragments of transgenic DNA had been detected in the study it should also be noted that the World Health Organisation

(1993) concluded that there is no inherent risk in consuming DNA, including that from GM crops. The basis of their conclusion was that mammals have always consumed significant quantities of DNA from a wide variety of sources, including plants, animals, bacteria, parasites and viruses. This is also not considered as a safety issue by regulatory agencies in US, Canada, Japan or the EU.

Scientific studies have also demonstrated that transgenic DNA and/ or protein expressed in GM crops are not detectable in the raw food products derived from animals fed with transgenic crops (Beever and Kemp, 2000; Beever and Phipps, 2001). Animal digestive systems rapidly degrade DNA and proteins. Moreover, studies have shown that ensiling and feed processing results in DNA fragmentation (Phipps, 2002). Based on the safety analyses required for GM crops, consumption of milk, meat, and eggs derived from farm animals fed with transgenic crops could be considered as safe as traditional counterparts.

Pigs

Piva *et al.,* (2001) reported that the performance of the pigs was significantly higher when offered the GM based diet and this was attributed to the fact that GM insect protected maize grain had significantly lower mycotoxin content when compared with the conventional maize grain (Table 2).

Table 2 : Nutritional Equivalence comparing conventional and Bt maize grain.

Pigs: at 2 locations	Conventional maize	Bt maize grain	Significance
Daily gain g/d	375	396	P<0.05
Final Live-weight	22.0	22.6	P< 0.05

Chickens

A control parental line (DK580), a glyphosate-tolerant line (GA21/ DK580) and five commercial varieties of corn were evaluated with 560 growing broiler chickens (80/treatment) in a 39-d growth trial (Sidhu *et al.,* 2000). Growth, feed efficiency, feed efficiency adjusted for feed consumption of dead chickens, and fat pad weights were not different for chickens fed the control or glyphosate-tolerant corn (Table 3). Likewise, these same measurements were not different for chickens fed the glyphosate-tolerant corn and the population mean for chickens fed the five commercial corn varieties. However, the performance of the chicken was significantly higher when offered the GM based diet and this was attributed to the fact that GM insect protected maize grain had significantly lower mycotoxin content when compared with the conventional maize grain Piva *et al.,* (2001).

Table 3 : Performance of chicken fed a control parental line (DK580) a glycophosphate tolerant line (GA21/DK580) and five commercial lines of corns.

Item	Mean BW (kg)	Feed efficiency	Feed efficiency (Adj)	Fat pad Wt
Males				
Control	1.945	1.662	1.629	1.638
GA21/DK580	2.013	1.750	1.646	1.775
Commercial lines	1.947	1.699	1.650	1.625
Females				
Control	1.859	1.779	1.721	2.114
GA21/DK580	1.885	1.781	1.749	2.085
Commercial lines	1.874	1.789	1.744	2.119

Future prospect of GM Feeds in livestock's

GM feed ingredients in near future will benefit livestock with improved feed qualities, availability of feeds per hectares of crops production. Further GM feed crops will have enhanced nutritional characteristics (Thomas and Bradford, 2001; Aumaitre *et al.,* 2002). The researchers are aimed at manipulating levels of proteins, amino acids, oil, and carbohydrates in major feed crops. GM crops being developed with improved nutritional characteristics include higher concentration of methionine and increased protein digestibility of lupins, increased lysine content in canola and soybean, increased levels of free and protein-bound threonine in lucerne, and reduced phytate content in corn grain (Aumaitre *et al.,* 2002). Researchers are also looking for ways to improve digestibility of wheat, rye or barley. Many of these biotech crops are already under field evaluation. The use of insect protected corn is already improving feed quality by decreasing mycotoxin contamination. The presence of mycotoxins in feed grains or ingredients makes them unfit for animal (or human) consumption and can cause serious health risk. GM crops expressing antigens from various microbes are also being developed. Edible vaccines delivered via feeds have the potential to control economically important diseases in livestock.

Conclusion

In the advancing modern age, agricultural production systems cannot be continued in their present form and there is a need for new technology that can produce more food of improved nutritional value and can reduce crop losses readily encountered by pest attack. On the other hand safety assurance of GM crops is mandatory to introduce as foods or feeds for human or livestock respectively. However, safety assessments conducted with plant biotech products provide equal or greater assurance of safety for food and feed use. There is a growing body of scientifically valid information that indicates safety of GM crops for feeds use in livestock's. The GM crops have directly benefited livestock production through safer and more abundant feeds source. Further GM crops with enhanced output traits have the profound effect of improving animal productivity and performance. These innovations will pave a way to provide sufficient foods or feeds to the growing world human and livestock's population.

However, genetic modification is not a panacea for improvement in agriculture, but it is one tool in an increasingly hungry world and technology in all its forms that makes agriculture productive.

References

Agnihotri, A. and Kaushik, N., (1998). Transgressive segregation and selection of erucic acid strain from intergeneric crosses of *Brassica*. *Indian J. plant genetic resources*, **11**(2): 251-255.

Artim, L., Charlton, S., Dana, G., Faust, M., Glenn, K., Hartnell, G., Hunst, P., Jennings, J., Shillito, R. (2001). Animal Performance Trials with Bt Maize. Proceedings of the 4th Pacific Rim Conference - Biotechnology of Bacillus thuringiensis and Its Environmental Impact, Australian National University, Canberra, Australia, Nov **11-15**: 246-253.

Aumaitre, A., K. Aulrich, A. Chesson, G. Flachowsky and G. Piva. (2002). New feeds from genetically modified plants: Substantial equivalence, digestibility, and safety for animals and the food chain. *Livestock Production Science*, **74**(3):223-238.

Beever, D.E. and C.F. Kemp. (2000). Safety issues associated with the DNA in animal feed derived from genetically modified crops: A review of scientific and regulatory procedures. Nutrition Abstracts and Reviews, Series B: *Livestock Feeds and Feeding,***70**(3):175-182.

Beever, D.E. and R.H. Phipps. (2001). The fate of plant DNA and novel proteins in feeds for farm livestock: A United Kingdom perspective. *Journal of Animal Science*, **79**(E. Suppl.):E290-E295.

Bell, J.M. (1984). Nutrients and toxicants in rapeseed meal - a review. *J. Anim. Sci.* **58**: 996-1010.

Chesson, A., Flachowsky, G. (2003). Transgenic Plants in Poultry Nutrition. *World's Poultry Science Journal.* **59**: 201-208.

Clark, J.H. and I.R. Ipharranguerre. (2001). Livestock performance: feeding biotech crops. *Journal of Dairy Science,* **84**(E. Suppl.):E9-E18.

Castillo, A.R., Gallardo, M.R., Maciel, M., Giordano, J. M., Conti, G.A., Gaggiotti, M.C., Quaino, O., Gianni, C. and Hartnell, G.F. 2004.Effects of feeding rations with genetically modified whole cottonseed to lactating dairy cows. *J. Dairy Sci.***87**:1778-1785.

Cromwell, G. L.. Lindemann, M. D Randolph, J. H. Parker, G. R. Coffey, R. D. Laurent, K. M. Armstrong, C. L. Mikel, W. B. Stanisiewski E. P. and G. F. Hartnell, (2002). Soybean meal from roundup ready or conventional soybeans in diets for growing-finishing swine*J Anim Sci.* **80**:708-715.

Delgado, C., M. Rosegrant, H. Steinfeld, S. Ehui and C. Courbois. (1999). Livestock to 2020: The next food revolution. Food, Agriculture, and the Environment Discussion Paper 28, International Food Policy Research Institute, Washington, DC; Food and Agriculture Organization, Rome, Italy; International Livestock Research Institute, Nairobi, Kenya.

Faust,M.A., (2000). Livestock products Corn composition and detection of transgenic DNA/proteins. In: Symposium held inconjunction with

American Dairy Science Association and American Society of Animal Science Meeting. Baltimore, USA, July 2000.

Flachowsky, G., Aulrich, K., (2001). Nutritional assessment of feeds from genetically modified organism. J. Anim. Feed Sci. **10**:181–194.

Folmer, J., Grant, R. and Beck, J. (2001). Use of Bt corn silage and grain by lactating dairy cattle.

Dairy Report (2001-2002) University of Nebraska, Lincoln.

Gilbert, R. (2000). Future economic benefits of GMOs in animal feeds with reference to soybeans and corn. Agriwatch Livestock Newsletter, 27 September 2000.

Iwarsson, K. and P.O. Nilsson, (1973). The effect of feeding rapeseed meal on thyroid function and morphology in growing Bulls. *Acta Vet. Scand.* **14**: 620-629.

K.K. Singhal (2008). Effect of feeding cottonseed produced from Bt cotton cultivar on feed intake, production and composition of milk in dairy cows.

Kuiper, H. A., G. A. Kleter, H. P. J. M. Noteborn, and E. J. Kok. (2001). Assessment of the food safety issues related to genetically modified foods. *Plant J.* **27**: 503–528.

MacKenzie, D. and M. McLean. (2002). Who's afraid of GM feed? Feed Mix, **10**(3):16-19.

Munkvold, G. P., R. L. Hellmich, and W. B. Showers. (1997). Reduced *Fusarium* ear rot and symptomless infection in kernels of maize genetically engineered for European corn borer resistance. *Phytopathology* **87**:1071-1077

Munkvold, G. P., R. L. Hellmich, and L. G. Rice. (1999). Comparison of fumonisin concentrations in kernels of transgenic Bt maize hybrids and nontransgenic hybrids. *Plant Dis.*.**83**:130-138.

Organization for Economic Cooperation and Development (OECD). 1993. Safety Evaluation of Foods Derived from Modern Biotechnology. OECD, Paris, http://www.oecd.org/dataoecd/57/3/1946129.pdf (14 July 2004).

Organization for Economic Cooperation and Development (OECD). 1996. Biotechnology Regulatory Contacts in OECD Member Countries, http:/

/www.oecd.org/document/17/0,2340,en_2649_34385_1890001_1_1_1_1,00.html (1997).

Organization for Economic Cooperation and Development (OECD). 1998. Biotechnology Regulatory Contacts in OECD Member Countries, http://www.oecd.org/document/19/0,2340,en_2649_34385_,00.html.

Padgette S.R., Taylor N.B., Nida D.I., Bailey M.R., MacDonald J., Holden M.R., Fuchs R.L., (1996). The composition of glyphosate-tolerant soybean seed is equivalent to that of conventional soybeans. *J. Nutr.* **126**: 702-716.

Pailan, G.H. and K.K. Singhal, (1997). Effect of dietary glucosinolates on nutrient utilization, milk yield and blood constituents of lactating goats. *Small Ruminants Research*. **71**; 31-37

Papas, A., J.R. Ingalls, and L.D. Campbell. (1979). Studies on the effects of rapeseed meal on thyroid status of cattle, glucosinolate and iodine content of milk and other parameters. *J. Nutr*. **109**: 1129 -1139.

Piva, G., M. Morlacchini, A. Pietri, F. Rossi, and A. Prandini. (2001). Growth performance of broilers fed insect- protected (MON810) or near isogenic control corn. Poult. Sci. 80(Suppl. 1):320. (Abstr)

Piva, G., Morlacchini, M., Pietri, A., Piva, A. and Casadei, G. (2001). Performance of weaned piglets fed insect-protected - MON 810 - or near isogenic corn. *Journal Animal Science* **79**. Suppl. 1: 106. Abstract 441.

Phipps, R.H. (2002). Safety of food products derived from livestock receiving GM feed ingredients. International Conference on Food and Feed Safety. Doha, Qatar, September.

Rosegrant, M.W., M.S. Paisner, S. Meijer and J. Witcover. (2001-2020) Global Food Outlook: Trends, Alternatives, and Choices. International Food Policy Research Institute, Washington, DC.

Singhal ,K. K., (1986). Oil seed cake for live stock feedin,. National dairy development institute, karnal, India, publication no. 220.

Sidhu, R. S., B. G. Hammond, R. L. Fuchs, J. Mutz, L. R. Holden, B. George, and T. Olson. (2000). Glyphosate-tolerant corn: The composition and feeding value of grain from glyphosate-tolerant corn is equivalent to that of conventional corn (Zea mays L.). *J. Agric. Food Chem*. **48** : 2305-2312.

TERI (The Energy and Resources Institute) (2003). NATP on sustainable management of plant biodiversity: chemical characterization of rapeseed-mustard for glucosinolates content. TERI. Project report no. 993364, submitted to national bureau of plant genetic resources, ICAR, New Delhi, pp.58.

Thomas, B.R. and K.J. Bradford. (2001). Crop biotechnology: Feeds for livestock. http://sbc.ucdavis.edu/outreach/abc/livestock_feeds_abc.htm.

World Health Organisation, (1993). Principles of the Safety Assessment of Food Additives and Contaminants in Food, Environmental Health Criteria 70.World Health Organisation, Geneva, Switzerland.

Zhang, B. H. and Feng, R., (2000). *Cotton Resistance to Insects and Insect-Resistant Cotton*, China*Agricultural Science and Technology Press*, Beijing.

❑❑❑

Chapter 6

A Brief Overview of Mastitis and Other Infectious Diseases of Cattle in India having Public Health Concern

BLESSA SAILO [1] AND SANDIP CHAKRABARTY [2]
[1] Scientist, ICAR complex, North Eastern Hill Region (Manipur sub center), India
[2] MVSc, Bangalore Veterinary College

Bovine Mastitis

Introduction

Mastitis (Mast: breast, itis: inflammation) is defined as an inflammatory reaction of udder tissue to bacterial, chemical, thermal or mechanical injury. Mastitis may be either infectious caused by microbial organisms or non-infectious resulting from physical injury to the gland. The inflammatory response consists of an increase in blood proteins and white blood cells in the mammary tissue and the milk. The purpose of the response is to destroy the irritant, repair the damaged-tissue and return the udder to normal function. It is the most costly disease of dairy cattle. About 40% of the cows are infected in an average of two quarters in an herd without an effective mastitis control programme. Reduced milk production accounts for about 70% of the total loss associated with mastitis.

Impact of mastitis in Indian condition

Bovine mastitis is the most complex disease condition mainly because of multiple causative agents, poor understanding of the early immune response and complexities associated with mammary epithelial cell damage by both the agents and the host factors. Decreased milk production accounts for approximately 70% of the total cost of mastitis. Though, India is the largest milk producer but per capita production is less than half of the world average. Additionally, the poor understanding of the underlying phenomenon in sub clinical state of the infection complicates the therapeutic interventions. It has been observed that about 95% of intramammary infections are caused by Streptococcus agalactiae, Staphylococcus aureus, Streptococcus dysgalactiae, Streptococcus uberis, and Escherichia coli. The remaining 5% are caused by other organisms. Very comprehensive knowledge of most predominant causative agents and their molecular signature defining the genetic diversity is not available. Further, understanding the disease process emphasizing the contribution of agent and host in the context of modern developments in biological sciences is of paramount importance and this has not been attempted in India, so far. The studies elsewhere in the world have started giving specific insights but the overall understanding is still very poor to arrive at definitive intervention/ mitigating strategies. It is in this backdrop, the objectives set out in this research programme will enable us to understand the critical aspects of host-microbe interaction. It will also provide an insight into the intricacies of the progression of the disease so that strategies for rapid diagnosis of sub clinical mastitis can be evolved. In addition, interventions for mitigation of sub clinical and clinical mastitis can be designed and validated for reducing the enormous economic loss incurred due to this disease worldwide. Pathogens invading the mammary gland cause a complex signalling network that activates the early immune defence and leads to inflammation. To examine the importance of mammary epithelial cells in these regulatory pathways, the prime focus is on MEC to infection by specific pathogen. The innate immune response is characterized by the induction of pro-inflammatory cytokines, as well as increases in other accessory proteins that facilitate host recognition and elimination of the pathogens. Thus, the objectives formulated will facilitate better understanding of disease process so that interventions can be designed. But if in case these objectives are not met, the need of the hour will be overlooked and as a consequences, the dairy industry in particular and Indian agriculture as a whole will continue to suffer from huge economic losses. Further, quality of milk has also a great bearing on Public health and such threat to the society will prevail, which will hinder the progress towards making the Indian agriculture globally competitive and ensuring food and nutritional security.

In India, mastitis is a disease with a great economic impact and the estimated loss due to this disease is around Rs. 16,702 millions per annum. Sub clinical mastitis has been found more important in India (varying from 10-50% in cows and 5-20% in buffaloes) than clinical mastitis (1-10%). The incidence was highest in purebred Holsteins and Jerseys and lowest in local cattle and buffaloes. The monsoon season is more suitable for the occurrence of sub clinical mastitis than summer or winter. Prevalence increases with higher lactation number and animals in 4th-5th month of lactation are more susceptible (59.49%) with the characteristic feature of hind quarters being more affected (56.52%) than fore quarters (43.47%). The factors like herd size, agro climatic conditions of the region, variations in socio-cultural practices, milk marketing, literacy level of the animal owner, system of feeding, and management are important in affecting the incidence of sub clinical mastitis. Comparison of efficacy of different diagnostic techniques for sub clinical mastitis, such as Modified California Mastitis Test (MCMT), bromo thymol blue (BTB), modified whiteside test, trypsin inhibition test, milk pH and electric conductivity indicate that MCMT is most sensitive and specific test.

The antimicrobial susceptibility tests have revealed on various occasions that most of the bacterial strains, whether gram positive, gram negative or mixed, isolated from subclinical mastitis milk samples, are highly sensitive to enrofloxacin, least sensitive to oxytetracycline and ampicillin and resistant to streptomycin. The therapy with enrofloxacin and nimesulide are more efficacious in treating sub clinical mastitis in milch cows. Identification of a mastitis pathogen is required for infection study. More than 99% of the mastitis pathogens are bacteria. Sub clinical mastitis is more important in India (varying from 10–50% in cows) than clinical mastitis (1–10%) (Joshi and Gokhale 2006). A number of reports on isolation and characterization of pathogens with special reference to plethora of bacterial species including even Rhodococcus equi (Wani *et al.,* 2003), Mycoplasma (Sanjeev Kumar *et al.,* 2005) and fungi (Reports of Monga 1969) are available but few reports of involvement of viruses in mastitis are available so far. Staphylococcus aureus, Streptococcal species and E. coli constituted major reported pathogens causing mastitis. Several studies have been conducted in the country from time to time to assess the chemotherapeutic efficacy of antimicrobials, relatedness among various isolates of pathogens like Staph aureus and E. coli by analysing the dendogram based antibiogram profile and to justify the application of advanced molecular tools like ERIC-PCR in the diagnosis of mastitis.

The IL-2 and IFN-gamma have been expressed in normal healthy cows and diseased cows after Azadirachta indica treatment, whereas both the cytokines could not be expressed in cows treated with antibiotic and in untreated diseased cows. The results of the present study indicated anti inflammatory, antibacterial and immunomodulatory potential of the herb (De and Mukherjee 2008). Enhancement of antioxidative and cellular defense and reduction of somatic cell count in the mastitic animals treated with enrofloxacin, vitamin E and selenium as compared to the enrofloxacin treatment alone has been demonstrated in experiments in bovine species with subclinical mastitis (Mukherjee 2008).

Development of the disease

Mastitis begins after the infectious agent like bacteria pass through the teat duct and enter the cisternal area. Invasion of the teat usually occurs during milking. Organisms present in the milk or at the teat end enter the teat canal and cistern when there is admission of undesired air in the milking unit. After milking, the teat canal remains dilated for 1-2 hours while the canal of a damaged teat may remain partially open permanently. This makes it easier for organisms from the environment or those found on injured skin to enter the teat canal. Adherence of bacteria to tissues lining cisterns and ducts may prevent flushing-out during milking thus helping in establishment of infections. Bacteria eventually enter the glandular tissues where they affect alveolar cells.

Toxins produced by bacteria cause either death or damage to milk-secreting epithelial cells and these cells produce substances that circulate in the blood stream and increase blood vessel permeability. This allows leukocytes to move from the blood into the alveolus where they function by engulfing the pathogen.

Etiological agents

Bacteria are by far the most common cause of mastitis. The most common bacteria include Streptococcus agalactiae and Staphylococcus aureus. S. agalactiae is the most common cause of sub clinical mastitis but rarely cause acute mastitis. The organism lives inside the cow's udder and survives only for a short time outside the mammary gland. It spreads primarily during milking via the milking machine, and contaminated hands and clothings. S. aureus lives inside and outside the udder on the teat skin. The microorganism can cause both clinical and sub-clinical mastitis and spreads the same way as Strep. agalactiae. Environmental mastitis is mainly caused by organisms like Escherichia coli, Strep. uberis, Mycoplasma, Klebsiella sp. and Pseudomonas aeruginosa that do not normally live in the skin or udder but enter the teat canal when the cow comes in contact with the contaminated environment (Harmon 1994). Yeast like Candida sp. can also cause mastitis wherein overuse of antibiotics and poor sanitation contribute to mastitis. Apart from the above organisms, Arcanobacterium pyogenes and Corynebacterium bovis are associated with Summer mastitis.

Types of mastitis

Mastitis can be broadly classified as Contagious and environmental mastitis. Contagious mastitis is caused by bacteria that live on the skin of the teat and inside the udder and can be transmitted from one cow to another during milking. The causal agents of environmental mastitis (like E.coli as mentioned under the heading Etiological agents) are normally found in feces bedding materials, and feed. Cases of environmental mastitis rarely exceed 10% of the total mastitis cases in the herd.

Contagious mastitis can be divided into three groups viz., clinical, sub-clinical and chronic. Clinical mastitis is characterized by the presence of gross inflammation signs. Three types of clinical mastitis exist viz., per-acute, acute and sub-acute. Per-acute form is characterized by gross inflammation, disrupted functions like reduction in milk yield and changes in milk composition and systemic signs like fever, depression, shivering, loss of appetite and loss of weight. Acute mastitis is similar to the per-acute form but with lesser systemic signs. In case of sub-acute mastitis, the inflammatory signs are minimal and no visible systemic signs are observed. Sub-clinical mastitis is characterized by change in milk composition with no signs of gross inflammation or milk abnormalities. Chronic mastitis for the most part exist as sub-clinical but may exhibit periodical flare-ups in the form of sub-acute or acute form and last for a short period of time. The chronic form may also continue from one lactation to another.

Table 1 : Changes in milk composition associated with mastitis

Components	Normal milk	Mastitic milk	% of normal
Solid-not-fat	8.98	8.80	99
Fat	35.0	3.20	91
Lactose	4.90	4.40	90
Total protein	3.61	3.56	99
Total casein	2.80	2.30	82
Whey protein	0.80	1.30	162
Serum albumin	0.02	0.07	350
Lactoferrin	0.02	0.10	500
Immunoglobulins	0.10	0.60	600
Sodium	0.06	0.105	184
Chloride	0.09	0.147	161
Potassium	0.17	0.157	91
Calcium	0.12	0.04	33

Symptoms

Inflammation is characterized by gross abnormalities in the udder viz., swelling, heat, redness, pain. Persisting inflammation leads to tissue damage and replacement of secretory tissues with of the udder with non-productive connective tissues. Abnormalities in milk may include flakes, clots or a watery appearance. The flakes in the milk are congealed leukocytes, secretory cells and protein. Ultimately, there is decreased milk yield.

Important Diagnostic approaches

Handling of milk sample

The quality of samples for mastitis diagnosis is in many respects more critical than that for many other diseases. Aseptic technique in sample collection for bacterial culturing is an absolute necessity as these same organisms have the potential to cause the disease. Contaminated samples may lead to misdiagnosis. Labelling of samples prior to sampling and including date, farm, cow number and quarter are essential. Using a hand or dry paper towel, loose dirt, bed¬ding and hair from the underside of udder and teats should be brushed. Discarding a few streams of milk from the quarter and observing milk and udder for signs of clinical mastitis along with predipping all quarters in an effective germicidal predip product and allowing 30 seconds of contact time is of utmost importance. To collect individual quarter samples, sampling should be started from the closest teat towards the teats on the far side of the udder i,e. the reverse order from cleaning. To collect the sample, the cap should be removed from the tube or vial but touching the inner surface of the cap should be avoided. The open end of the cap should always be kept in a downward position. Maintaining the tube or vial at approximately a 45-degree angle while taking the sample is important. Samples should be properly packaged and kept cold at a temperature of less than 40ºF or kept frozen during shipping (Waldner 1999).

Cow side testing

California Mastitis Test (CMT)

The California Mastitis Test is a simple, inexpensive, rapid screening test for mastitis. The test is based upon the amount of cellular nuclear protein present in the milk sample. Since inflammatory cells associated with mastitis are the predominant cell type present in milk the CMT reflects the SCC level quite accurately and is a reliable indicator of the severity of infection. It is important to understand that a certain percent (around 10-20%) of cows sampled for bacterial culture based on CMT score will have no growth. This is due to a number of factors including short lived infections that have been cleared by the cow or infections that are characterized by intermittent shedding of bacteria like Strep. agalactiae, Staph aureus and mycoplasma. The test is appropriate for cow-side evaluation of udder health. The CMT can also be used to evaluate composite milk samples as well as bulk tank milk. In a crisis situation where a herd is at risk of losing it market or quality premiums the test can be used to screen animals or quarters to withhold from the bulk tank. Test criteria for commingled milk are less severe than that for quarter samples because of the dilution effect of milk from normal quarters or cows. It is noteworthy that the value of CMT evaluation of bulk milk decreases as herd size increases.

Table 2 : Relationship between CMT scores and somatic cell count (Jasper 1967)

CMT score	Somatic cell range
N	0-200,000
T	200,000-400,000
1	400,000-1,200,000
2	1,200,000-5,000,000
3	Over 5,000,000

R-Mastitest

R-Mastitest is used as indirect test for cow's mastitis diagnosis and it is based on the principle of Californian Mastitis Test (Sargeant *et al.,* 2001). The reagent used in R-Mastitest consists of sodium laurilsulphate, nonylphenol, polyethylene glycol 4000 and bromcresole purple as pH indicator. Homonigenized milk with an equal amount of reagent results in dissolution and rupture of cell and nuclear membranes. This leads to the release of DNA molecules, which will connect and form a gel. The consistency of gel resulted increases as the number of neutrophiles, macrophages, lymphocytes and epithelial cells (in other words the somatic cells) are higher in a mammary quarter.

Electrical conductivity

Mastitic milk has a higher electrical conductivity than normal milk due to tissue damage and the subsequent increase in Sodium and Chloride ions in milk. Conductivity sensors are being incorporated in many new automated milking systems. The change in electrical conductivity is one of the earliest manifestations associated with new infections making the routine early detection and recording of possible mastitis cases possible. But the greatest problem associated with this new technology is the sensitivity and specificity of electrical conductivity between herds. However, recent advances in determining herd specific conductivity threshold levels have increased the value of this screening method in many herds. The Mast-O-Test method is a specialised test based on the relationship between milk electrical conductivity and its salt and lactose content (Musser *et al.,* 1998).

Laboratory tests

Bulk tank Somatic cell counts (BTSCC)

Bulk tank somatic cell counts (BTSCC) are to be reported to dairy producers on a routine basis usually on bimonthly basis as a measure of milk quality. BTSCC scores can also be used to monitor the level of udder health. In general BTSCC less than 200,000 cells/ml indicate a minimal level of infection, however a series of BTSCC's over 500,000 cells/ml indicate a problem with sub clinical or chronic infection. As the BTSCC is a function of both the quarter infection rate and the severity of infections, attempts to predict the infection status from a single BTSCC proves to be unsuccessful. This is particularly true in case of small herds where an elevated tank count may be the result of exceptionally high counts in a few cows or from a general elevation of counts from many cows.

Individual Cow Somatic Cell Counts (SCC)

The most important factor affecting the SCC of milk from a quarter, cow or herd is the infection status of the quarter (Schepers *et al.,* 1997). Individual cow somatic cell counts are the product of the SCC measurement of all milk from all four quarters and the level of production of the individual quarters. Average SCC for uninfected quarters range between 170,000 to 214,000 cells/ml or a geometric mean of 106,000 cells/ml. Somatic cell response of infected cows will depend somewhat on the pathogen present. Minor pathogens such as C. bovis and coagulase-negative Staphylococcus average 227,000 cells/ml when all age groups are considered. Animals infected with major pathogens like Streptococcus agalactiae, Staphylococcus aureus or Environmental Streptococci produce average counts greater than 600,000 cells/ml. The number of infected quarters as well as the total milk production become important factors in being able to accurately classify a cow as infected by means of SCC. The dilution effect of normal milk can mask infection.

Table 3 : Relationship between SCC linear score (LS) and Somatic cell count (SCC) range (Shook and Seaman 1983)

LS	SCC range
0	0-18,999
1	19,000-35,999
2	36,000-71,999
3	72,000-1,41,999
4	1,42,000-2,83,999
5	2,84,000-5,65,999
6	5,66,000-1,130,999
7	1,131,000-2,262,999
8	2,263,000-4,523,999
9	4,524,000 - >9,999,999

Linear score

Official test scores of somatic cell counts are typically reported as Log linear scores of the raw SCC. Log linear scores provide a more accurate and direct measure of milk losses associated with increasing

SCC. The average LS give a less distorted and more accurate picture of a lactation than does the average raw SCC. For these reasons linear score is used most frequently when analyzing and graphing SCC data.

Culturing of milk

Culturing milk from the bulk tank, individual quarter or cow, groups or categories of cows helps in adding an additional dimension to evaluating udder health and mastitis control programs especially when the information is combined with SCC or clinical mastitis data. Routine milk cultures is an important component of any mastitis control program. Sampling the bulk tank milk (BTC) is a simple, inexpensive means of determining the presence of mastitis pathogens in a herd. This culturing method is best suited for the identification of contagious mastitis pathogens and for monitoring the presence of pathogens over time. BTC from herds with a low prevalence of infection with a specific organism, especially contagious pathogens like Staphylococcus aureus, Streptococcus agalactiae and Mycoplasma spp. may not always indicate the presence of those pathogens. Hence, BTC results should always be considered when collected as a series of tests over a given period of time.

Individual animal culture

Individual animal cultures provide another method of diagnosing mastitis. Cultures alone provide an indication of the possible pathogen involved. However the possibility of a false positive result due to contamination of the sample with organisms present in the teat canal, teat skin or environmental contamination of the sample can affect test specificity. Individual cow culture results become much more meaningful when combined with SCC results. Using SCC to select cows at high risk to be sampled for milk culture ensures a relatively good predictive value for the culture results. Using two tests simultaneously to evaluate animals increases the sensitivity but causes slight decrease in the specificity. Predictive value (PV) of a test is defined as the proportion of infected animals among those that are test positive. The predictive value of any given test is a function of the test specificity, sensitivity as well as the prevalence of the disease in the herd. The predictive value of a test decreases as the prevalence of the disease decreases within the herd. When applied to SCC and milk cultures the specificity of culture results improves as the SCC threshold increases. In most herd investigations using an LS of 4.0 (SCC = 200,000 cells) provides approximately 70 to 80 % sensitivity and specificity.

Capture immunoassays using monoclonal antibodies

A direct capture enzyme-linked immunosorbent assay (ELISA) can be used to measure elevated polymorphonuclear granulocyte (PMN) antigens using horseradish peroxidase conjugated rabbit polyclonal anti-PMN antisera and a monoclonal antibody specific for PMN cells. Optical densities obtained in the ELISA are useful to predict the cell counts of milk samples (O'Sullivan *et al.,* 1992).

DNA approach

DNA amplification of the target pathogen by PCR even though is more expensive than culture method, but the efficiency and accuracy of pathogen identification is high. Million to billion fold amplification of the targeted DNA sequence can be achieved by using pathogen specific probes. For instances, the use of Pathoproof Mastitis PCR assay for amplification of the staphylococcal beta-lactamase gene has gained popularity in recent years. By this assay pathogen identification can be done within 4 hours. The use of diagnostic kits like MasTest helps in health monitoring and breeding for mastitis resistance as such kits can detect pathogen related variability in heritability and aids in selection of marker genes. Automated quantitative real time PCR (qRT-PCR) is fast, accurate and helps in quantitative detection of pathogen upto species level (Report of Bredbacka and co-workers).

Computerized herd record analysis

Use of computerized herd record analysis programs such as Dairy Comp 305 allows management to be more proactive in dealing with udder health and issues involving milk quality. Monitoring can also serve as a motivational tool and marketing device for quality milk technical services. Producers who enter other disease and health data into Dairy Comp can also evaluate the incidence and prevalence of clinical mastitis the possible interaction other health problems such as metabolic disease, DA, retained placenta etc with udder health (NYSCHAP reports).

Prevention and control

Measures aiming at preventing new cases of mastitis from occurring include breeding, improvement of milking hygiene, implementation of post-milking teat disinfection, regular controls of the milking equipment, implementation of milking order, and improvement of bedding material. Antibiotic treatment protocols, dry cow therapy, and culling regimes are examples of actions that are taken in order to limit the impact of mastitis once it has occurred (Nielsen 2009). When a herd problem is faced, the proper sampling method to employ should be determined in accordance with the history of the herd and the urgency of the situation. Herds with a history characteristic of contagious mastitis such as a steady rise in BTSCC or those highly suspect of having contagious mastitis may benefit from an initial bulk tank culture. Any herd known to have contagious mastitis caused by Staphylococcus aureus, Streptococcus agalactiae or Mycoplasma spp. with an interest to eliminate the infection from the herd must have a whole herd survey. A whole herd survey provides an estimate of infection prevalence or an inventory of mastitis pathogens in a herd. A single survey provides an excellent estimation of the herd prevalence rate of specific pathogens. When elimination of a contagious pathogen such as Strep. agalactiae becomes a herd goal, frequent herd surveys become necessary. Success of such a program is heavily dependant upon accurate identification of infected animals so that infection can be contained by means of segregation of infected animals at milking time as well as effective treatment of the infected animals. A delay in the time interval between surveys will allow the infection to spread, hindering the eradication process and increasing the associated costs. Such principle of conducting quick and accurate survey apply to the contagious pathogens such as Staphylococcus aureus and Mycoplasma spp. Mycoplasma infections are untreatable. Infected cows can remain infected for life, become intermittent shedders and are a constant source of new infections. Culling infected cows provides the most effective means of infection control. Staph aureus infection is also very difficult to cure. This is particularly true for treatment during lactation. Treatment at dry off offers a greater opportunity to eliminate infections but Staph aureus infection too frequently carry through to the next lactation. Producers with relatively low levels of infection or low BTSCC can be benefitted from milk cultures of problem animals. Milk cultures based on stage of lactation or history can provide valuable information concerning pathogen prevalence, monitoring the effectiveness of control programs or treatment protocols and is used to identify risk factors for new infection. For instance, the dry period is a known risk factor for new infections by environmental pathogens. Environmental Streptococci and coliform infections are 2 to 12 time more likely to occur during the dry period than lactation. To provide a better understanding of the new infection rate during the dry period a producer can use linear score to select cows for sampling and possible treatment. A producer not taking advantage of computerized herd record analysis data can use CMT results to reach similar conclusions. A similar testing method can be used to samples cows at dry off to identify quarters of the infected cows, evaluate the effectiveness of dry cow treatment or use selective dry cow therapy. Culturing clinical quarters can provide valuable information concerning pathogen prevalence and provide a more logical means of selecting appropriate treatment protocols. When used in conjunction with SCC and other production parameters the data can provide valuable insight for identifying risk factors such as stage of lactation, low SCC, parity, or production group and provide a basis for evaluating the effectiveness of vaccination programs or treatment methods.

Considering that most cows in a herd are of second or later parities and that SCC is highest in multiparous cows, the majority of the production loss caused by mastitis is likely to be experienced by multiparous cows. Thus, special emphasis should be put on reducing the incidence of mastitis in multiparous cows. This can be attempted by enhanced mastitis control in primiparous cows because cows that have suffered from mastitis are more likely to develop subsequent cases. Attention should be paid to cows in early and late stages of lactation. During these periods, the incidence of mastitis is highest and yield losses are most severe, but, by taking proper actions, unnecessary milk loss can be avoided.

The frequency of mastitis in the dairy cow population can also be decreased by breeding for cows with better ability to resist udder disease. Udder health is unfavourably genetically correlated with milk yield (Carlen *et al.,* 2004), and selecting only for increased production, which traditionally has been the focus of dairy cattle breeding. This can be counteracted by applying a broad breeding goal which includes not only production traits, but functional traits such as mastitis resistance. The genetic progress in a trait is partly determined by the relative weight put on it in the total merit index of bulls. In order to assign proper economic weight to mastitis resistance, accurate estimates of the economic loss caused by mastitis are necessary (Carlen 2008).

Understanding the genetics of mastitis susceptibility

Breeding for resistance to udder pathogens is an important tool. Periparturient mastitis susceptibility is related to the generalized immune suppression taking place from approximately 1 week prepartum to approximately 1 week postpartum. Thus, it is necessary to identify the genes responsible for such condition. Genetic selection against periparturient mastitis susceptibility may be the best long-term approach. The global gene expression changes occurring in bovine blood leukocytes around parturition has been done by cDNA microarray analysis. However, it has not been determined which population of leukocytes are affected or what factors of parturition cause the repression of the leukocyte genes (altogether 18 genes have been identified by microarray experiment). A majority of them showed high DNA sequence homology to genes that are needed for normal cell functions (Burton *et al.,* 2003). The new finding in the gene expression studies include the identification of the gene that produces a protein that is naturally present in cows' milk and blood plasma but in an amount too small to have any therapeutic effect. The recombinant protein, named CD14 binds to and neutralizes endotoxins that are made by bacteria causing mastitis. Studies are now being conducted to support the new hypothesis that cows genetically engineered to produce higher than normal amounts of CD14 can get protection from infection as well. Moreover, numerous experiments have identified different QTL regions in cattle. These QTLs envelop large chromosomal regions on average spreading from 10 to 40 cM which involve hundreds or thousands of genes. The goal of QTL analysis is identification of the causal gene itself. Besides QTLs, a large number of genetic polymorphisms within the causal gene regions or genetic markers associated with mastitis traits have also been identified in cattle by microarray analysis. New knowledge regarding the genetics of mastitis susceptibility ultimately helps in the development of novel management strategies.

Infectious diseases of cattle in India having public health concern

Introduction

Changes in pathogen and host ecology are primarily responsible for the majority of diseases transmissible to human. Ecological changes embrace a number of processes under the same umbrella viz., changes in agricultural practices, urbanisation, globalisation or climate change (Schrag and Wiener 1995). Factors associated with the emergence of pathogens in human and domestic animals like cattle have been explored from time to time (Daszak *et al.,* 2001). In recent years, it seems that humans have probably been responsible for many zoonotic diseases through creating and maintaining the conditions for existing pathogens to enter, persist and develop in new host populations (Dobson and Foufopulos 2001). Disease emergence is the result of two sequential processes viz., the adaptation of a pathogen to a new host and the spread of the pathogen into the new population. These pathogens have adverse effects on indigenous fauna and are considered to be one of the most important causes of the global biodiversity crisis. They are also recognised as a clear threat to ecosystems, habitats or species, with severe economic and environmental consequences (CBD 2003). Such pathogens are of great public health concern and the diseases caused by them may be acquired or spread in a variety of ways viz., through the air (aerosol), by direct contact, by contact with an inanimate object that harbors the disease (fomite transmission), by oral ingestion, and by insect transmission. The present chapter gives a brief outline of such diseases.

Anthrax

Anthrax is a naturally occurring disease with worldwide distribution. It is caused by Bacillus anthracis, a spore-forming bacteria that can remain dormant in the soil for many years. The organism can bloom and contaminate surface soil and grass after periods of wet, cool weather, followed by several weeks of hot, dry conditions. The anthrax zones are found in areas wherein the soil is heavily contaminated with anthrax spores. Such conditions include soil rich in organic matter (pH <6.0) and dramatic changes in climate, such as abundant rainfall following a prolonged drought. Anthrax can infect humans in three ways which have been discussed in chapter 1 and so also will be discussed now. Skin anthrax also known as the cutaneous anthrax may be contracted by handling contaminated hair, wool, hides, flesh, blood, or feces of infected animals, as well as through manufactured products such as bone meal. Infection is introduced through scratches, abrasions, or wounds of the skin. It is the mildest form of human anthrax. Symptoms include itching, rash and lesions near the site of infection. With proper treatment, skin anthrax is fatal in less than 1% of all cases. Approximately 95% of human anthrax infections are cutaneous infections. Gastrointestinal anthrax is contracted by orally ingesting anthrax spores, usually by eating insufficiently cooked infected meat. Symptoms include cramps, diarrhoea, and fever. Gastrointestinal anthrax infections are unlikely from handling contaminated packages. Inhalation anthrax is contracted by inhaling spores directly into the lungs. Such infections normally occur among workers handling infected animal hides. After an incubation period of one to seven days, the infected individual gradually develops flu-like symptoms such as fever, malaise, fatigue, cough, and mild chest discomfort. This mild disease can progress rapidly to respiratory distress and shock in two to four days, followed by a range of more severe symptoms such as difficulty in breathing and exhaustion. Under natural conditions, inhaled anthrax is exceedingly rare (Friedlander 1999). In case of human anthrax, post exposure prophylaxis may be achieved with oral ciprofloxacin (500 mg twice a day) or doxycycline (100 mg twice a day). Biothrax vaccine has been developed in USA which is an alum precipitated toxoid containing protective antigen treated with formalin. Chemoprophylaxis is best continued until the exposed person has received at least three doses of vaccine for a minimum period of 4 weeks). If vaccine is unavailable, chemoprophylaxis has to be continued for 8 weeks (Friedlanders *et al.,* 1993).

Brucellosis

Brucella organisms can be present in birthing tissues or fluids (aborted fetuses, fetal fluids, placentas, and vaginal discharges), and also in milk, urine, blood, and semen. Transmission among cattle is through ingestion of birthing fluids and milk and in utero. Most infections in humans are associated with drinking or eating unpasteurized milk products. Much of the milk which is consumed is rendered safe by pasteurisation or boiling, but cheese is preferably prepared from untreated milk. During the course of cheese manufacture, any Brucella present in the milk become trapped in the clot and thus concentrated in the cheese, although bacteria may subsequentiy be inactivated by manufacturing or ripening processes. Cream and ice cream prepared from milk also possess risk of transmission (Flores-Castro and Baer 1980). Handling infected aborted fetuses or afterbirth is another com¬mon means of human infection due to the entry of the organisms through cuts in the skin and the mucous membranes of the eye and mouth.

Common symptoms in humans are undulating fever, weakness, headache, joint pain along with night sweats. Human brucellosis can be prevented by avoiding drinking of unpasteurised/untreated dairy products and wearing gloves when handling reproductive tissues. Hands should be washed after touching or handling animals.

Escherichia coli infection

Escherichia coli (E. coli) are bacteria normally found in the intestines of human and cattle. However, some strains cause a severe, often bloody, diarrhea in humans. Cattle act as the carriers of the bacteria and humans be¬come infected by ingesting contaminated food or water, especially undercooked groun beef (Bielaszewska *et al.,* 1997). Humans may also become infected after handling or being exposed to feces of a carrier animal. Person-to-person transmission can occur by lack of good hand washing following diaper changes. E. coli O157: H7 is a particularly virulent strain of E. coli that causes asymptomatic infection in cattle in most of the instances but has the potential of causing abdominal cramping and bloody diarrhea in human occasionally life threatening kidney disease and a hemolytic uremic syndrome in children and elderly person. Prevention focuses on hand washing and proper food hygiene. Hands and all cooking equipment should be washed with soap and hot water after touching or handling raw meat. Meats should be thawed in the refrigerator, and ground beef should be cooked until it reaches an internal temperature of 165°F and the juices run clear. Eating undercooked meat or drinking unpasteurised milk should be avoided. Hands should be washed after handling animals and eating or drinking around animals should be avoided. Day-care facilities should wash toys frequently, and individuals with diarrhea should avoid swim¬ming in public areas. In outbreaks of other primary transmission routes, secondary cases occur, which emphasizes the importance of educating caretakers to avoid direct contact with faecal matter and to apply stringent hand washing rules. Virulent O157 antigen-specific phages can play a role in effective biocontrol of the infection in animals and fresh food stuffs without compromising the viability of other normal flora or food quality (Kudva *et al.,* 1999).

Salmonellosis

Salmonella spp. are shed in the feces of infected animals. Many animals are susceptible to Salmonella including cattle. Infection occurs as a result of the ingestion of contaminated feed, water, or grass. The bacterium can live for months to years in the environment, especially in wet and warm conditions. People acquire Salmonella from undercooked contaminated meat or unpas¬teurized milk products. If hands are not washed after direct contact with infected feces, then accidental ingestion of bacteria can occur. Humans may develop diarrhea, abdominal cramping and fever which can be very severe. For primary screening of human cases (especially paratyphoid caused by S. paratyphi), Widal test is most frequently employed which is a slide agglutination test for detecting somatic A and B antigens followed by detection of flagellar H antigen. Drugs like chloramphenicol and imepenam are used for treatment of human infection but there is chance of multiple drug resistance and thus the antibiogram profiles needed to be studied first. Regular microbiological monitoring of the slaughter house by products, insect control, preventing the pet animals from consuming inedible offals are among some of the basic preventive measures. Meat should be adequately cooked and proper food handling hygiene should be used. Hands should always be washed after touching or working with animals. Strategies for preventing infection by raw milk cheeses should be aimed at both producers and consumers. Strict and carefully planned hazard analysis critical control point procedures should be developed and implemented for unpasteurised dairy products (Robinson and Jones 1981). As part of this procedure any batch of cheese made from raw milk should be closely monitored for Salmonella and distribution should be avoided until known to be clear. Producers should also report positive results of end production internal sampling to public health authorities. Consumers particularly those susceptible to infectious diseases (eg., infants, elderly people and immunocompromised patients) should also be warned that a nil risk cannot be warranted for raw milk products.

Tuberculosis (T.B)

Humans may acquire M. bovis, the causative agent of bovine tuberculosis from unpasteurized dairy products and can develop symptoms involving the lungs, kidneys, spine, or brain. Infected individuals have a persistent cough and often cough up blood. There is increasing need of screening human patients for T.B by performing Mantoux test which is an intradermal skin test that detects skin thickness of 5 mm or more 48-72 hours following the administration of liquid tuberculin. Several drugs like streptomycin, para-amino-salicilic acid, isoniazid and rifampicin are available for treatment of T.B in human. The cornerstone of treatment for TB lies in the use of combination of drugs like isoniazid, rifampicin, pyrazinamide and ethambutol for two months followed by isoniazid and rifampicin alone for a further four months. The patient is considered cured at six months, even though there is still a relapse rate of 2 to 3%. For latent tuberculosis, the standard treatment is six to nine months of isoniazid alone (Grange and Zumla

2002). Prevention is by avoiding consumption of unpasteurized dairy products.

Leptospirosis

Leptospirosis is a zoonoses which can be transmitted from animal to animal and animal to human. The original natural carrier for serovar icterohaemorrhagiae is rodent. Cattle acts as the rervoir host for Lepto serovar hardjo-bovis. Transmission of the organism to human can occur through skin abrasions and mucous membranes by contact with urine or tissues of animals infected with leptospirosis. Apart from this, ingestion and inhalation can also transmit the disease. Human infections vary from asymptomatic to severe. Many cases are mild or asymptomatic and remain unrecognized. Usually, it occurs as a biphasic illness in human. The first phase, called the acute or septicemic phase begins abruptly and lasts approximately a week. This phase is characterized by nonspecific signs including fever, chills, headache and conjunctival suffusion. Myalgia, which typically affects the back, thighs or calves, is often severe. Occasionally, a transient skin rash occurs. Other symptoms may include weakness, photophobia, lymphadenopathy, abdominal pain, nausea, vomiting, a sore throat, cough, chest pain and hemoptysis. Mental confusion, neck stiffness and other signs of aseptic meningitis are also characteristics of this phase. Jaundice can be seen in more severe infections. These symptoms last for approximately 4 to 9 days, then are typically followed by a 1 to 3 day period during which the temperature drops and the symptoms disappear. The second phase of leptospirosis, called the immune phase, is characterized by the development of anti-Leptospira antibodies, and the excretion of the organisms in the urine. This phase can last up to 30 days or more, but does not develop in all patients. During the immune phase, the patient becomes ill again. Non-specific fever and myalgia are seen during the first phase recur but may be less severe than in the first stage of disease. Two forms of disease, icteric and anicteric, are seen. Most infections are of the anicteric form. The most important symptoms in this form are associated with aseptic meningitis. A severe headache, stiff neck and other meningeal symptoms occur in approximately half of all patients, and usually last a few days. Occasionally, these signs may be present for up to two weeks. Less common symptoms include cranial nerve paralysis, encephalitis, confusion and changes in consciousness. Deaths are rare in the typical anicteric form. However, a syndrome of fatal pulmonary hemorrhage, without jaundice, has recently been reported. The icteric form is more severe. It occurs in 5-10% of all patients, is often rapidly progressive, and may be associated with multiorgan failure. The most commonly involved organ systems are the liver, kidneys and central nervous system (CNS). In the icteric form, there may be no period of improvement between the septicemic and immune phases. Jaundice can be severe and may give the skin an orange tone, but it is not usually associated with severe hepatic necrosis. Acute renal failure occurs in 16-40% of cases (OIE 2005). Some patients also have pulmonary symptoms, with clinical signs ranging from cough, dyspnea, chest pain, and mild to severe hemoptysis, to adult respiratory distress syndrome. Cardiac involvement can result in congestive heart failure, myocarditis and pericarditis. Hemorrhages may also be seen; epistaxis, petechiae, purpura and ecchymoses are the most common signs, but severe gastrointestinal bleeding, adrenal or subarachnoid hemorrhage, and pulmonary hemorrhages can occur. Rare complications include stroke, rhabdomyolysis, thrombotic thrombocytopenic purpura, acute acalculous cholecystitis, erythema nodosum, aortic stenosis, Kawasaki syndrome, reactive arthritis, epididymitis, nerve palsy, male hypogonadism, Guillain-Barre´ syndrome and cerebral arteritis. Deaths can occur from kidney failure, cardiac involvement. pulmonary hemorrhage or other serious organ dysfunction. Convalescence from the icteric form may take 1-2 months. Although jaundice can persist for weeks, liver function returns to normal after recovery, and hepatic disease is rarely the cause of death. Most patients also recover kidney function. Anterior uveitis occurs up to a year after recovery. Iridocyclitis and chorioretinitis can also be complications, and may persist for years. Abortions, fetal death, and rare congenital infections in newborns are among the problems associated with reproductive failure. Abortions can occur at any time, including the convalescent period. As far as the human to human transmission is concerned, it occurs rarely. Leptospira organisms are found in the urine during the second (immune) phase of the disease.

Most people excrete these bacteria for 60 days or less, but shedding for months or years have also been documented.

Microscopic agglutination test (MAT) is the gold standard test, but it is complicated and less sensitive compared to newer tests like IgM ELISA and SAT. As IgM ELISA and Slide agglutination tests (SAT) are simple, sensitive tests which measure IgM antibodies, they are currently used to diagnose leptospirosis at a very early stage instead of MAT. Single sample is adequate for these two tests. The IgM ELISA test is particularly useful in making an early diagnosis, as it is positive as early as 2 days into illness, a time when the clinical manifestation may be nonspecific. It was found to be 100% sensitive and 93% specific in one study (Kaur *et al.,* 2003). Dot-ELISA and dip-stick methods for detecting IgM antibodies are newer screening methods. Faine has evolved a criteria for diagnosis of leptospirosis on the basis of clinical (A), epidemiological (B) and laboratory data (C) respectively. A presumptive diagnosis of leptospirosis may be made if: (i) Parts A and B score = 26 or more (Part C laboratory report is usually not available before fifth day of illness. Thus, it is mainly a clinical and epidemiologic diagnosis during early part of disease) (ii) Part A+B+C = 25 or more. A score between 20 and 25 is suggestive of a possible but unconfirmed diagnosis of leptospirosis (Faine 1982). Modification on Faine's criteria include local factor like rainfall and newer investigations in the total scoring. As per this, epidemiological and laboratory criteria (Parts B and C) are modified only. No modification is made in the clinical criteria (Part A) (Shiva Kumar and Shareek 2004). Severe leptospirosis in human can be treated with antibiotics like doxycycline. ampicillin, amoxicillin, penicillin and erythromycin. Doxycycline may be used for short time prophylaxis. The control of infection in goats and especially pet animals reduces the risk of human disease, but the existence of wild life reservoirs complicate the disease prevention. Rodent control is important in preventing human infections, particularly in urban areas (Russel 1994). Personal hygiene and protective clothing are important preventative measures in high risk occupations. Gloves and face shields can help in preventing infections while working with infected animals or tissues. Rubber boots can decrease the risk of infection in sewer workers and agricultural workers who come in contact with urine-contaminated water.

Listeriosis

Listeriosis, caused by Listeria monocytogenes (Lm) is transmitted from cattle to human either directly through contact with infected animals or indirectly via milk, cheese or meat (Washington state department of health 2002). Listeriosis in humans is seen primarily in pregnant women, newborns, elderly, and immunosuppressed (e.g. transplant recipients or AIDS patients). A small population (5-10 %) may act as asymptomatic carriers harboring the organism in their feces or vagina. Disease in adult humans is commonly of the encephalitic or septicemic/visceral form (Working group on zoonoses 2002). The most common treatment is administration of antibiotics like oxytetracycline or penicillin G. Good hygiene and sanitation on the farm is of utmost importance to prevent the spread of the disease to human population. Whenever possible, people at risk for listeriosis should avoid the consumption of foods associated with listeriosis as mentioned earlier. The risk group also need to adhere strictly to the food label directions for storage and "use by" information. It is virtually impossible to provide Listeria-free food products because L. monocytogenes infects many animal species with many infections being inapparent, and most importantly the bacterium can survive and grow at refrigeration temperature levels. Other means of prevention include thoroughly cooking raw meats, proper hygiene during food preparation and consuming only pasteurized dairy products. Humans at risk should also avoid contact with animals that have aborted as well as with aborted materials like placenta and fetuses on the farm. Moreover, livestock and crop producers can also help to control the spread of L. monocytogenes by avoiding the use of untreated manure on vegetable crops.

Ringworm

Ringworm is a skin infection in human that can be transmitted from cattle and the species of importance is T. verrucosum. People are infected with ringworm through direct contact with infected animals. In humans, ringworm forms itchy areas on the skin that are round and irritated.

Treatment helps to limit the spread of the disease to other susceptible person. Topical iodine compounds (5%), chlorhexidine (2%), lime sulphur (2%-5%), and topical antifungal medications are useful for local treatment of lesions. Some severe cases require administration of medications. People treating animals should always wear gloves and protective clothing to prevent from getting this disease (www.ext.vt.edu). Proper cleaning and disinfection of clippers, blankets and other equipment with antiseptic solutions along with good sanitation practices of animal handlers help control the spread of this disease.

Rabies

People contract rabies through exposure to infected saliva in open wounds or mucous membranes of eyes, nose and mouth. This can occur during examination or treatment of infected cattle. However, other contacts such as petting a rabid animal or contact with the blood, urine or faeces of a rabid animal do not constitute an exposure and is not an indication for prophylaxis (Afshar 1979). After the first exposure, there is acute incubation phase of the disease during which itching and discomfort occur at the site of bite wound. It has a sensation of needle pricking the skin. In addition, the person may develop fever and a headache. These symptoms may last from 2 days to weeks. This is followed by another incubation period. The National Institute of Health (NIH) suggests that the average latent incubation phase may vary from 3 to 7 weeks although a period extending to about 10 years is also reported. Thereafter, there is development of symptoms like anxiety, delirium, drooling of saliva, convulsion, hallucination, loss of sensation in an area of the body, insomnia and swallowing difficulty. When these symptoms develop, the person is likely to die. When people develop clinical rabies, the best treatment is supportive care. Healthcare providers do not generally recommend routine pre-exposure prophylaxis with the rabies vaccine in other situations. Healthcare providers administer pre-exposure prophylaxis with the rabies vaccine for several reasons. First, it simplifies therapy by eliminating the need for human rabies immune globulin (HRIG), and decreases the number of rabies vaccine doses needed. Second, it may enhance immunity in people whose post-exposure rabies treatment might be delayed. Finally, it may provide protection to people with inapparent exposures to rabies. Pre-exposure treatment with the rabies vaccine consists of three doses of rabies vaccine given on days 0, 7, and 21 or 28. Doctors use post-exposure prophylaxis (rabies treatment) with the rabies vaccine for people possibly exposed to a rabid animal. Post-exposure treatment for rabies should begin as soon as possible after an exposure. Physicians should evaluate each possible exposure to rabies and, as necessary, consult with local or state public health officials regarding the need for rabies prophylaxis. Post-exposure rabies treatment consists of a regimen of one dose of rabies immune globulin and five doses of rabies vaccine given over a 28-day period. Rabies immune globulin and the first dose of rabies vaccine should be given as soon as possible after exposure. Additional doses of rabies vaccine should be given on days 3, 7, 14, and 28 after the first vaccination. The rabies vaccine works by stimulating a person's immune system to produce antibodies that neutralize the virus. The person develops a protective immune response before the virus reaches the brain and begins to actively replicate. Older rabies vaccines required painful, daily injections in the abdomen, for up to three weeks, and they could produce severe side effects. Current rabies vaccines are relatively painless and are given in arm. Newer rabies vaccines in use today also cause fewer adverse reactions. Possible side effects of the rabies vaccine can include low-grade fever, pain, redness, swelling or itching at the injection site, headache, nausea, abdominal pain, muscle aches and dizziness (US Department of Health and Human Services 2009). Transmission of the virus in unpasteurised cow's milk is theoretically possible. The risk can be defined better if samples of milk and mammary tissues are collected from rabid animal and assayed for the presence, infectivity and viability of the rabies virus. Regardless of the amount of viavle rabies virus that may be shed in cow's milk, the theoretical risk of transmission of rabies via this route can be eliminated if all dairy products are pasteurized before consumption (National Association of State Public Health Veterinarians 1999).

Rabies can also spread to the existing cattle population from wild life reservoirs. In a cooperative program involving the USDA and the CDC, animals such as raccoons, coyotes, foxes, and skunks are vaccinated orally in certain areas of USA where rabid wildlife are frequently found. The oral rabies vaccine is hidden in a bait of fishmeal or other food. The baits are dropped by airplanes into rural areas and spread by hand in urban and suburban areas. But this approach is not feasible in developing countries like India and further studies are required in this aspect.

Fascioliasis

Studies carried out in recent years have shown human fascioliasis to be an important public health problem (Chen and Mott 1990). Fascioliasis in human have been reported particularly from the north-eastern part of the country (Narain *et al.,* 1997). Human F. hepatica infection is determined by the presence of the intermediate snail hosts, domestic herbivorous animals, climatic conditions and the dietary habits of man. Cattle are considered as the predominant animal reservoir. The mode of transmission is the faecal–oral route. Parasite eggs are passed in the faeces of infected animals or humans, thereby contaminating water where they develop within snails. The snails release mature larvae that attach to vegetation and encyst as metacercariae. A person typically becomes infected by ingesting encysted metacercariae attached to aquatic or semi-aquatic plants. Evidence also indicates that infection may occur by drinking water contaminated with floating metacercariae and by ingesting metacercariae attached to the surface of food or kitchen utensils washed with water contaminated with floated metacercariae. Fascioliasis is a serious medical condition due to the size of the parasite. After an incubation phase lasting days to a couple of months, human fascioliasis can be distinguished by an acute and a chronic phase. The acute phase is characterized by the migration of immature worms through the liver and the symptoms are related to haemorrhage and inflammation and are usually severe, including fever, abdominal pain, respiratory disturbances and skin rashes. The chronic phase starts when the worms reach the bile ducts but in such cases, the symptoms are non-specific and usually mild. However, progressive inflammation leads to fibrosis and thickening of the walls of the ducts and gallbladder that eventually may result in progressive blockage due to parasites, parasite fragments or debris. In this case, biliary colic pain is a characteristic symptom.

Chronic infections may result in biliary cirrhosis with scarring and fibrosis of the liver and growth deficiencies. Ultrasonography in addition to ELISA and Western Blot analysis of the parasitic antigen aid to diagnosis of human fascioliasis. False fasciolosis (pseudofasciolosis) refers to the presence of eggs in the stool not because of an actual infection but due to recent ingestion of infected livers containing eggs. This situation with its potential for misdiagnosis can be avoided by having the patient follow a liver-free diet several days before a repeat stool examination (Hillyer 1999). Single dose of triclabendazole (Fasinax@10 mg/kg body weight) is the most common drug of choice against human fascioliasis. The drug is active against both immature and adult parasites with high cure rates (O'Brien 1998).

References

Afshar, A. A. (1979). A review of non-bite transmission of rabies virus infection. British Vet J., 135: 142-148.

Bielaszewska, M., Janda, J., Blahova, K., Minarikova, H., Jikova, E., Karmali, M. A., Laubova, J., Sikulova, J., Preston, M. A, Khakhria, R., Karch, H., Klazarova, H. and Nyc, O. (1997). Human Escherichia coli O157: H7 infection associated with the consumption of unpasteurized goat's milk. Am. Pub. Health. Assoc., 119: 299-305.

Bredbacka, P., Salmikivi, L. and Koskinen, M. T. Next-day results in bovine mastitis diagnostics using DNA technology and electronic reporting. Finnzymes Diagnostics.

Burton, J. L., Madsen, S. A., Yao, J., Sipkovsky, S. S. and Coussens, P. M. (2003). An immunogenomics approach to understanding periparturient immunosupression and mastitis susceptibility in dairy cows. Acta. Vet. Scand., 98: 71-88.

Carlen, E. (2008). Genetic evaluation of clinical mastitis in dairy cattle. Doctoral Thesis. Swedish University of Agricultural Sciences, Uppsala, Sweden.

Carlen, E., Strandberg, E. and Roth, A. (2004). Genetic parameters for clinical mastitis, somatic cell scores, and production in the first three lactations of Swedish Holstein cows. J. Dairy Sci., 87(9): 3062-3070.

Chen, M.G. and Mott, K.E. (1990). Progress in assessment of morbidity due to Fasciola hepatica infection: a review of recent literature. Trop. Dis. Bull., 87: R1–R38.

Dairy Cattle Production 342-450A. Mastitis in dairy cows. Faculty of Agricultural and Environmental Sciences. Department of Animal Science. Mac Donald Campus of Mac Gill University.

Daszak, P., Cunningham, A. A. and Hyatt, A. D. (2001). Anthropogenic environmental change and the emergence of infectious disease in wildlife. Acta trop., 78(2): 103-116.

De, U. K. and Mukherjee, R. (2008). Anti-inflammatory and respiratory burst activity of Azadirachta indica during acute bovine mastitis. Ind. J. Anim. Sci., 79(2): 32-34.

Dobson, A. and Foufopoulos J. (2001). Emerging infectious pathogens of wildlife. Philos. Trans. roy. Soc. Lond., B, biol. Sci., 356(1411): 1001-1012.

Faine, S. (1982). Guidelines for the control of leptospirosis. WHO Offset Publication No. 67, Geneva.

Flores-Castro, R. and Baer, G. M. (1980). Brucellosis (Brucella melitensis), Zoonotic implications. In: CRC Handbook series in Zoonoses, Section A: Bacterial, Rickettsial and Mycotic diseases, CRC Press Inc., Boca Raton, F. L. 195.

Friedlander, A. M. (1999). Clinical aspects, diagnosis and treatment of anthrax. J. Appl. Microbiol., 87: 303.

Friedlander, A. M., Welkos, S. L., Pitt, M. L. M., Ezzell, J. W., Worsham, P. L. and Rose, K. J. (1993). Postexposure prophylaxis against experimental inhalation anthrax. J. Infect. Dis., 167: 1239-42.

Grange, J.M. and Zumla, A. (2002). The global emergency of tuberculosis: what is the cause? J. Royal Soc. Promot. Health., 122(2): 78–81.

Harmon, R. J. (1994). Mastitis and genetic evaluation for somatic cell count – Physiology of mastitis and factors affecting somatic cell counts. J. Dairy. Sci., 77(7): 2103-2112.

Hillyer, G. V. (1999). Immunodiagnosis of human and animal fascilosis. In: Dalton, J. P. Fasciolosis. Wallingford, Oxon, U. K. CABI Pub. pp. 435-447.

http://www.bvs.sld.cu.

http://www.dpi.vic.gov.au.

Jasper, D. E. (1967). Proceedings of National Masitis Council (adapted).

Joshi, S. and Gokhale, S. (2006). Status of mastitis as an emerging diseases in improved and periurban dairy farms in India. Annals of The New York Acad. Sci., doi: 10.1196/annals.1373.007.

Kaur, I. R., Sachdeva, R., Arora, V. and Talwar, V. (2003). Preliminary survey of leptospirosis among febrile patients from urban slums of East Delhi. J. Assoc. Physic. Ind., 51: 249-51.

Kudva, I. T., Jelacic, S., Tarr, P. I., Youderian, P. and Hovde, C. J. (1999). Biocontrol of Escerichiacoli O157 with O157 specific bacteriophages. Appl. Environ. Microbiol., 65(9): 3767-3773.

Monga, D. P. (1969). Studies on mastitis due to fungi and mycoplasma in domestic animals. Under the guidance of Dr. D. S. Kalra.

Mukherjee, R. (2008). Selenium and Vitamin E increases polymorphonuclear cell phagocytosis and anti-oxidant levels during acute mastitis in riverine buffaloes. Vet. Res. Commun., 32(4): 305-313.

Musser, J. M. B., Anderson, K. L. and Caballero, M. (1998). Evaluation of a hand-held electrical conductivity meter for detection of subclinical mastitis in cattle. Am. J. Vet. Res., 59: 1087-1091.

Narain, K., Biswas, D., Rajguru, S. K. and Mahanta, J. (1997). Human distomatosis due to Ffasciola hepatica infection in Assam, India. J. Commun. Dis., 29(2): 161-165.

National Association of State Public Health Veteriarians, Inc. (1999). Compendium of animal rabies control. J. Am. Vet. Med. Assoc., 214: 198-202.

New York State Cattle Health Assurance Programme (NYSCHAP) Veterinary Resource. Diagnosis of mastitis and diagnostic methods for investigating udder health problems.

Nielsen, C. (2009). Economic impact of mastitis in dairy cows. Doctoral Thesis. Swedish University of Agricultural Sciences, Uppsala, Sweden.

O'Brien, D. J. (1998). Fasciolosis: a threat to livestock. Irish Vet. J., 51: 539–541.

O'Sullivan, C. A., Joyce, P. J., Sloan, T. and Shattock, A. G. (1992). Capture immunoassay for the diagnosis of bovine mastitis using a monoclonal antibody to polymorphonuclear granulocytes. J. Dairy Res., 59(2): 123-133.

OIE. (2005). The centre for food security and public health. Leptospirosis. pp 1-9.

Robinson, D. A. and Jones, D. M. (1981). Milk-borne campylobacter infection. BMJ., 282:1374-1376.

Russell, L. (1994). Leptospirosis. Scientific meeting for leptospirosis. pp. 5-7.

Sanjeev Kumar, M., Murag, S. and Hari Babu, Y. (2005). Biochemical and immunological identification of mycoplasma isolates from bovine mastitis. SRDDL, Institute of Animal Health and Veterinary Biologicals, Hebbal, Bangalore.

Sargeant, J. M., Leslie, K. E., Shirley, J. E., Pulkrabek, B. and Lim, G. H. (2001). Sensitivity and specificity of somatic cell count and California Masititis Test for identifying intramammary infection in early lactation. J. Dairy Sci., 84: 2018-2024.

Schepers, A. J., Lam, T. J. G. M., Schukken, Y. H., Wilmink, J. B. M. and Hanekamp, W. J. A. (1997). Estimation of variance components for somatic cell counts to determine thresholds for uninfected quarters. J. Dairy Sci., 80(8): 1833-1840.

Schrag, S. J. and Wiener, P. (1995). Emerging infectious disease: what are the relative roles of ecology and evolution. Trends Ecol. Evol., 10(8): 319-324.

Shiva Kumar, S. and Shareek, P. S. (2004). Diagnosis of leptospirosis utilizing modified Faine's criteria. J. Assoc. Physic. Ind., 52: 678-679.

Shook, G. and Seaman, A. (1983). JDS., 39(12).

United Nations Convention on Biological Diversity (CBD) (2003). Pilot Assessments: the ecological and socioeconomic impact of invasive alien species on island ecosystems. CBD, Montreal, pp. 38. Website: http://www.biodiv.org/doc/ref/alien/ias-inland-en.pdf.

US Department of Health and Human Services. (2009). Vaccine information statement. Centres for Disease Control and Prevention.

Waldner, D. N. (1999). Bovine mastitis: Milk sample collection and handling. Division of Agriculturl Sciences and Natural Resources. Oklahoma State University. Oklahoma Cooperative Extension Fact Sheets. http://osufacts.okstate.edu.

Wani, S. A., Bhat, M. A., Qureshi, S. and Bachh, A. S. (2003). Isolation of Rhodococcus equi from clinical bovine mastitis – A case report. Ind. J. Anim. Res., 37(1): 75-76.

Washington State Department of Health. (2002). Listeriosis. pp. 1-5.

Working Group on Zoonoses. (2002). Zoonotic Pathogens: Health Risks from Listeria. Federal Veterinary Office Magazine. pp. 14-15.

www.ext.vt.edu.

□□□

Chapter 7

Foot and Mouth Disease in Livestock and its Diagnosis

NEETA LONGJAM[1] AND A.K. SARMAH[2]

[1.] MVSc, [2.] Professor, Department of Veterinary Microbiology, College of Veterinary Science, Assam Agricultural University, Khanapara, Guwahati-781022, India

Introduction

Foot-and-mouth disease (FMD) is a highly contagious disease affecting artiodactylae, mostly cattle, swine, sheep, goats and many species of wild ungulates (Brooksby, 1982). It is recognized as a significant epidemic disease threatening the cattle industry since sixteen century and till date it is a major global animal health problem. The history of FMD may be traced to era of Hieronymous Fracastorius, a monk who described a disease outbreak in 1546 A.D. occurred in cattle near Verona, Italy (Fracastorius, 1546). Almost 400 years later, in 1897, Friedrich Loeffler and Paul Frosch demonstrated that a filterable agent is responsible for FMD (Loeffler and Frosch, 1897). This was the first demonstration that a disease of animal was caused by a filterable agent and ushered in the era of virology.

FMD generally involves mortality rates below 5%, but even so it is considered the most important disease of farm animals since it causes huge losses in terms of livestock productivity and trade. Although FMDV rarely causes death in adult animals, the virus can cause severe lesion in the myocardium of young animals, leading to high mortality rates

(Domingo *et al.*, 1990; Woobury *et al.*, 1995). The main constraints in controlling this disease and why it is considered as the most dreaded viral disease are its high contagiousness, wide geographical distribution, broad host range, ability to establish carrier status, antigenic diversity leading to poor cross immunity and relatively short duration of immunity. The Office Of International des Epizooties (OIE) ranks the disease first in its list A diseases and the virus as Risk Group 4 of transboundary importance (OIE, 2008a and 2009). Poor surveillance and diagnostic facilities as well as inadequate control programs are major problems in control of this disease in the country. FMD is still a leading cause of loss of livestock economy in India. Outbreaks are still being reported from time to time round the year (Tamilselvan *et al.*, 2009). Besides causing direct losses to livestock economy it also causes indirect losses in terms of severe trade restrictions, impact which may be higher than direct losses.

The etiological agent, foot-and-mouth disease virus (FMDV) is classified within the genus Aphthovirus in the family Picornaviridae (Racaniello, 2001). The virus exists in the form of seven serologically and genetically distinguishable types viz. O, A, C, Asia1, SAT1, SAT2 and SAT3, but a large number of subtypes have evolved within each serotype (Pereira, 1977). Serotype O and A reported in France by Valee and Caree (1922) and in 1926, Waldmann and Trautwein reported serotype C. Serotypes SAT1, SAT2 and SAT3 of FMDV was observed in sample collected from the FMD outbreak in South Africa (Brooksby, 1958). The seventh serotype, Asia 1 was reported from Pakistan (Brooksby and Roger, 1957).

FMDV is a single stranded (ss) positive sense RNA virus with the whole virus particles having sedimentation coefficient of 146S (Bachrach, 1968) and genome of ~8.5 Kb size. The genome is polyadenylated at 3' end and carries a small covalently linked protein, VPg at 5' end (Bachrach, 1968). The 5' untranslated region (UTR) contains a short fragment called S-fragment, a poly (C) tract followed by large (L) fragment of over 700 bases. Functionally, the genome can be categorized into three main regions: a) 5' non-coding regulatory region, b) Polyprotein coding region (subdivided into L, P1, P2, and P3) and c) 3' non-coding regulatory region.

The translation initiation starts at two AUG codons separated by 84 nucleotides following the Internal Ribosome Entry Site (IRES) (Sangar *et al.,* 1987). The viral genome is translated as a single polyprotein, which is post-translationally cleaved by viral proteases (Ryan *et al.,* 1989) into four structural proteins (VP1, VP2, VP3 & VP4) and several non-structural proteins [(L, 2A, 2B, 2C, 3A, 3B, 3C & 3D) (Murphy *et al.,* 1999)]. The P1 region of genome encodes the 4 structural proteins VP1, VP2, VP3 and VP4 encoded by 1D, 1B, 1C and 1A genomic regions respectively (Bachrach, 1968). Sixty copies of each structural protein (VPl-4) assemble to form the capsid (Bachrach, 1968). Among which VP4 is internal whereas others are exposed on virion surface (Acharya *et al.,* 1989). The 3 surface exposed capsid proteins carry the neutralizing antigenic sites (Mateu, 1995). Among the 4 structural polypeptides, VP1 is the most immunogenic protein of FMDV (Logan *et al.,* 1993) having its G-H loop protruded from the surface (Bittle *et al.,* 1982; Pfaff *et al.,* 1982) and is maximally exposed on the capsid surface (Acharya *et al.,* 1989; Lea *et al.,* 1994) forming large part (54%) of virus surface (Morrel *et al.,* 1987).

In India Foot and mouth disease is endemic since many centuries. It is present almost in all parts of the country and occurs round the year. Approximately 470 million domestic livestock are susceptible to FMD apart from the free-living and captive wild ungulates. Out of the possible seven, only four serotypes, viz, =O', =A', =C' and Asia 1 were ever recorded in India. Serotype =C' too has not been recorded in the country since 1995. Currently more than 1500 outbreaks are being reported throughout the year, and more than 75% of the outbreaks are attributed to serotype =O', and the remaining 25 % of outbreaks are due to serotypes =A' and Asia1. This indicates that serotype =O' viruses are highly adapted to their host and environment to survive in the nature. The molecular epidemiological studies have established that the Pan-Asian strain is the major cause of outbreak of FMD involving serotype =O' in India

Although, the disease has been controlled successfully in many parts of the world by regular vaccination of susceptible animals and slaughtering of infected animals, no country has been considered safe, because of the highly contagious nature and rapid spread of the infection (Bruner and Gillespie, 1973). In India, FMD control is implemented by regular vaccination and for effective control, outbreaks should be detected at an early stage and persistent infections should also be recognized to prevent further transmittance. These can be achieved when vaccination is regular and effective and when diagnostic tools available are of specific and sensitive at the same time rapid.

Lots of work has been carried out to develop and validate diagnostic tests in regard to this disease. Conventional techniques such as complement fixation test (CFT, Traub and Mohlmann, 1943), serum neutralization tests (SNT) (Rweyemamu *et al.,* 1978) and enzyme linked immunosorbent assay (ELISA) (Have *et al.,* 1983) are still in use for the routine detection of FMDV in clinical samples. Of late, ELISA has largely replaced the use of CFT due to its sensitivity, specificity and ability to deal with large number of samples. On the other hand CFT also has the disadvantage of anti-complementary factor in some antigen and pro complementary factors in sera of some species of animals. Generally, sandwhich ELISA is carried for detection of specific FMDV antigens in epithelial tissue suspensions which is usually accompanied by concurrent cell culture isolation and the application of ELISA to any samples showing a cytopathogenic effect (Ferris and Dawson, 1988). Virus isolation in primary cultures is laborious, expensive and requires days/weeks (cell passages) before the results are obtained (Vangrysperre and De Clercq, 1996). However, with the introduction of molecular techniques in the field of diagnosis, several techniques based on viral genome detection such as hybridization using DNA probes (Rossi *et al.,*1988) and the advent of Polymerase Chain Reaction (PCR) technique in the recent past has led to development of several reverse transcription PCR (RT-PCR) procedures for specific detection of FMDV RNA (Meyer *et al.,* 1991; Laor *et al.,* 1992; Amaral-Doel *et al.,* 1993; Hofner *et al.,* 1993; Rodriguez *et al.,* 1994; Marquardt *et al.,* 1995). Because of the reported sensitivity and specificity, RT-PCR has been evaluated as a diagnostic tool for FMDV detection in parallel with ELISA and virus isolation (Reid *et al.,* 1998). Another form of PCR, multiplex PCR (mPCR), has also been evaluated for differentiating FMDV serotypes (Vangrysperre and De Clercq, 1996;

Callens and De Clercq 1997; Giridharan *et al.,* 2005) as well as for differential diagnosis with other vesicular diseases such as Vesicular' Stomatitis, Swine Vesicular Disease (Nuenz *et al.,* 1998). The most recent development in the field of diagnosis by nucleic acid detection is the use of thermal cyclers capable of measuring fluorogenic PCR amplification in real-time have become available, making precise quantitation of nucleic acids possible over a wide concentration range. The fluorogenic RT-PCR provides relatively fast result, enables a quantitative assessment to be made of virus amount and can handle more samples and/or replicates of samples in a single assay than the conventional RT-PCR procedure (Reid *et al.,* 2002).Therefore it is seen as a valuable tool to complement the routine diagnosis procedure for FMD virus diagnosis .

Currently, the FMD diagnosis in the country is being carried out using techniques developed at PD on FMD, Mukteswar which includes Virus isolation (VI), Sandwich-ELISA (S-ELISA),Liquid-Phase Blocking ELISA (LPBE), Multiplex-PCR (mPCR) and recently DIVA test which is an indirect ELISA for detection of antibody against non structural proteins. LPBE is being used for the detection of antibody titers against the FMD vaccinated animals. The S-ELISA is being used for the antigen detection using the material from the lesions but because of its low sensitivity currently mPCR is being used. The real time PCR based detection method is used in the many reference laboratories in the world for the purpose. In India recently, a Real-Time multiplex Taq-Man PCR was developed and is under evaluation for detection of FMDV in clinical samples (Tamil Selvan *et al.,*2009).

Etio-patho-epiemological Outlook

Foot-and-mouth disease virus (FMDV) was the first recognized viral pathogen (Loeffler and Frosch, 1898) and is the sole member of the genus Aphthovirus belonging to the Picornaviridae family. Seven immunologically different serotypes of the FMD virus are known, namely A, O, C, Asia-1, South-African Territories (SAT) -1, -2 and -3, which comprise more than 65 subtypes. Initially 2 types were named: type O for Oise in France and type A for Allemagne (Germany) (Vallee and Carre,

1922). Later type C was recognized as an additional type in Germany (Waldmann and Trautwein, 1926). Some 30 years later, work at Pirbright laboratory in England demonstrated 3 novel serotypes of FMDV in sample collected from the FMD outbreak in South Africa and called SAT1, SAT2 and SAT3 (Brooksby 1958). The seventh serotype, i.e. Asia 1 was first recognized in a sample from Pakistan (Brooksby and Roger, 1957).

The viral particle, or virion, contains a single-stranded RNA of positive polarity, approximately 8500 nucleotides long. It is an icosahedral particle with a smooth surface and a diameter of about 30 nm (Bachrach, 1968). The fine structure of the virus has been described by X-ray crystallography (Acharya *et al.,* 1989; Lee *et al.,* 1993; Jackson *et al.,* 2003). There are 60 copies of each of the structural protein VP1, VP2, VP3 and VP4. While the first three structural proteins (MW˜24 kDa) have surface components, the fourth (MW˜8.5 kDa) is internal. The virion is also usually composed of one or two units of VP0, the precursor of VP2 and VP4 (Acharya *et al.,* 1989; Domingo *et al.,* 1992.) The structural proteins, VP1-3 fold into an eight stranded wedge shaped ß-barrel which fits together to form the majority of the capsid structure (Acharya *et al.,* 1989). The three-dimensional structure of FMDV has revealed a prominent surface feature formed by the loop between the G and H strands of VP1. The VP4 protein is located inside the capsid (Belsham *et al.,* 1991). The strands of the ß-barrel of VP1-3 are connected by loops which form the outer surface of the virion (Jackson *et al.,* 2002). Unlike other picornaviruses, FMDV lacks a surface canyon or pit which is the receptor binding site for entero and cardioviruses (Belnap *et al.,* 2000). Another feature of the virion is the channel at the five fold axis which permits the entry of small molecules such as CsCl into the capsid resulting in FMDV having the highest buoyant density of the picornaviruses (Jackson *et al.,* 2003).

The main cell attachment site and the immunodominant region of FMDV are both located on a solvent exposed region at the surface of the virion, namely in trypsin-sensitive areas of VP1 (Laporte and Lenoir, 1973: Cavanagh *et al.,* 1977). Earlier serological studies showed that different serotypes of FMDV shared a highly variable region of VP1, comprising residues 135 to 155 (Strohmaier *et al.*, 1982), as one of the major antigenic sites of the virus.

3. Genome Organization of the Fmd Virus

The genome of FMDV is about 8.5 Kb in length enclosed within a protein capsid. It has four major parts: 5′ Untranslated region (5′UTR), Coding region, 3′ Untranslated region (3′UTR) and a poly ¯A? tail. The 5′UTR is linked with Vpg (3B) which serves as primer in replication. 5′UTR contains an S fragment at its 5′end which encompasses 360 bases, folds into long stem loop and plays a role in genome stability and the binding of protein involved in genome replication (Bunch *et al.*, 1994, Costa-Goami *et al.*, 1984). There are some evidences that length of this tract is associated with virulence and hence persistence (Harris and Brown 1977). After poly ¯C? tract, there is a series of RNA pseudo knot structures of unknown function (Grubmann and Baxt 2004). Downstream to the pseudo knot there is cis-acting replicative element (cre) (Mason *et al.*, 2002). The cre has conserved AAA sequences and is essential for genome replication (Mason *et al.*, 2002). Downstream to cre is internal ribosomal entering sites (IRES). The IRES has role in initiation of viral protein synthesis and shut down of host cell protein synthesis (Grubmann and Baxt, 2004). Due to the presence of IRES, picornaviruses are able to bind to ribosomes to initiate the protein synthesis.The picornaviruses have no 5′cap (7-methyguanosine), so IRES serves as ribosomal entering site (Jang *et al.*, 1988). The 3′UTR follows the ORF (open reading frame) termination codon and contains a short stretch of RNA which folds into a specific stem loop structures (Pilipenko *et al.*, 1992) followed by a poly ¯A? tract of variable length (Dorsch-Hasler *et al.*, 1975). This 3′UTR also serves as some functions in genome replication (Pilipenko *et al.*, 1996). 3′UTR is specific for each picornavirus. Poly ¯A? probably plays a role in FMDV translation (Lopez *et al.*, 2002) and replication (Herold *et al.*, 2001). The FMDV genome encodes a polyprotein from which four different structural and eight different non-structural proteins are formed by the viral proteases. After translation, the four primary cleavage products are formed: (i) the amino terminal L protease which cleaves at its own carboxy terminus, P1- 2A, (ii) the precursor of the capsid proteins (iii) 2BC and (iv) P3 which is cleave to make the NSPs (Belsham, 1993). FMDV has two proteinases. The NSP leader proteinses (Lpro) located in the N-terminal region of the polyprotein acts both intra and intermolecularly. This protease initiates cleavage by separating itself from P1, the precursor of the capsid protein and the remainder of the growing polypeptide chain (Ryan *et al.,* 1991). The 3C protease is responsible for the cleavage of P1 into 1AB (VP0), 1C (VP3) and 1D (VP1). The 1A/1B (VP4/VP2) cleavage occurs at the late stage in virus morphogenesis and is associated with maturation of capsid. The 2C/3A primary cleavage is cis and subsequent cleavage is also mediated by the 3Cpro and producing processing intermediates and mature proteins (Newman *et al.,* 1994). In addition to viral protein processing, the 3Cpro cleave the host cell protein histone H3 and may be involved with the shut down of host cell transcription (Capozzo *et al.,* 2002). The cleavage between 2A/2B junctions is mediated by 2A polypeptide separating itself and P1 away from 2BC/P3 (Belsham, 1993). This change is independent of both L and 3C. The FMDV 2A region is very short (about 18 amino acids) and together with the N-terminal residues of protein 2B, represents an autonomous element capable of mediating cleavage at its own C terminus (Donnelly *et al.,* 1997).

Foot-and-mouth disease (FMD) is an acute systemic infection affecting even-toed ungulates, both domesticated and wild, including cattle, swine, sheep and goats. Beside domesticated animals, other animals species affected with FMD includes elephant (Pyakural *et al.,* 1976; Sharma *et al.,* 1994), mithun (Dutta *et al.,* 1979; Verma *et al.,* 1997), yak (Barman *et al.,*1999), sambar, spotted deer and wild buffalo (Barman *et al.,* 1999; Vosloo *et al.,* 2002).

FMDV produces an acute, systemic vesicular disease, which requires a differential diagnosis from other vesicular diseases (Sutmoller, 1992). In natural infection, the main route of virus entry is the respiratory tract. The initial virus multiplication usually takes place in the pharynx epithelium, producing primary vesicles, or "aphthae" (Burrows *et al.,* 1981). The vesicles produced by FMDV generally affect cells from the epithelial stratum espinosum. The clinical outcome of the disease may vary among the host species considered and the infecting virus strain. In cattle and pigs, fever and viraemia usually start within 24–48 hr after epithelium infection, leading to viral spread into different organs and tissues and the production of secondary vesicles preferentially in the mouth and feet. The acute phase of disease lasts about 1 week and declines gradually coinciding with the emergence of a strong humoral response (Salt, 1993).The morbidity and mortality in FMD depends upon the breed and age of the animal where mortality in adult animals is very low (two per cent) in comparison to 20 per cent in young stock (Radostits *et al.,* 1994).The calves show prominent signs of myocarditis, whereas piglets manifest gastroenteritis (Buxton and Fraser, 1977). In sheep and goats, symptoms are frequently less severe and may make the detection of the disease difficult (Knowles *et al.,* 2001).

Asymptomatic, persistent infection can also be established in ruminants, during which infectious virus can be isolated from the oesophagus and throat fluids of the animals from a few weeks up to several years of the initial infection. There is epidemiological evidence to support the hypothesis that carrier animals may be the origin of outbreaks of acute disease when brought into contact with susceptible animals. This mode of transmission has been experimentally reproduced for serotype SAT isolates (Vosloo *et al.,* 1996).

FMD is a highly transmissible disease, and a limited number of infective particles can initiate host infection (Sellers, 1971). Contaminated animal products, non-susceptible animals, agricultural tools, people, vehicles and airborne transmission (Donaldson *et al.,* 1987) can contribute to the mechanical dissemination of FMDV. The epidemiology of FMD is complex, and it is affected by different viral, host and environmental factors, among them, variations in virus virulence (severity of lesions, amount and duration of virus release), particle stability in different microenvironments and chances of long-term persistence. FMDV multiplication and spread also depend on the host species, nutritional and immunological status, population density, animal movements and contacts between different domestic and wild host species and animals capable of mechanical dissemination of the virus (Nishiura *et al.,* 2010). The environment can provide geographical barriers to virus dissemination or, alternatively, can promote virus transmission when appropriate atmospheric conditions prevail. In this multifactorial scenario (Ferguson et.al.,2001; Sobrino and Domingo, 2001), the high potential for FMDV variation and adaptation has modelled complex evolutionary patterns that are being revealed by molecular epidemiology analyses, mostly based on nucleotide sequencing of capsid protein genes.

Of the different serotypes prevalent in India, type =O' has been found to be predominant over others types (Prasad, 1971; Tewari *et al.,* 1975; Prasad *et al.,* 1978; Ramakant *et al.,* 1980; Kumar *et al.,* 1983, 1994; Ahuja *et al.,* 1986,1996). Similarly in the North-Eastern region of India, the frequency of FMD is highest with type =O', which is always followed by other types including the type =Asia-1' (Dutta *et al.,* 1984; Sarma *et al.,* 1992).

The agro-climatic and socio-economic condition, mixed animal husbandry practices, unrestricted movement, trade among animals and porous international border provides a conductive epidemiology niche for the FMDV to flourish, mutate and persist over time and to affect the susceptible animal population (Rao, 1989; Mishra *et al.,* 1998).There are records of about 5,000 outbreaks to occur in India annually affecting nearly three lakh animals (Mukhopadhyay,1992) with an estimated staggering loss of Rs. 4,300 cores to the economy annually (Anon.,1991).The losses are mainly due to reduction in milk yield, draught power and breeding capabilities. In India where world's largest livestock populations exist, it is a leading cause of loss of livestock economy (direct and indirect losses) due to its endemic nature.

4. Diagnosis of FMD

The accurate diagnosis of infection with FMDV is of prime most importance for both control and eradication campaigns in FMD endemic areas and as a supportive measure to the stamping out policy in FMD free areas. The history of research and diagnosis in foot-and-mouth disease falls into several distinct areas. The search for experimental laboratory animals, producing the disease culminated in the demonstration by Waldmann and Pape (1920) the susceptibility of the guinea pig and the suckling mouse by Skinner in 1951. Early work by Hecke and the Maitlands in the early 1930s, followed by the crucial demonstration by Frenkel in 1947 that large amounts of the virus could be produced in surviving tongue epithelium, formed the basis for the vaccination programmes initiated in Europe in the 1950s (Fred Brown, 2003). The subsequent development of cell lines has brought a remarkable degree of sophistication to the study of virus growth. The recognition of more than one serotype has led to the development of various techniques for serotyping of the virus. As early as 1927, Bedson et al. found that two isolates of a serotype =A' virus could be differentiated by cross-neutralization tests (Bedson *et al.,* 1927). Earlier typing of FMDV was done by cross-immunity test in guinea pigs (Waldmann and Trautwein, 1926) and less frequently in cattle (Bachrach, 1968). As this test was time consuming, expensive and imprecise (Rweyemamu, 1982) different serological tests like complement fixation test (CFT), virus neutralization test (VNT) and enzyme linked immunosorbent assay (ELISA) were developed and the most recent is the development of molecular techniques, the polymerase chain reaction (PCR) method making diagnosis more rapid and precise.

4.1. Complement Fixation test (CFT)

In 1929, Ciuca was first to use CFT for typing antiserum and FMDV of guinea pig origin (Bachrach, 1968). Later, virus of bovine origin was successfully typed by CFT using guinea pig antiserum (Traub and Mohlman, 1943). Since then CFT has been used extensively for distinguishing different strains of FMDV (Traub and Mohalmann, 1946; Brooksby, 1952; Davie, 1964; Rweyemamu *et al.,* 1978; Ferris *et al.,* 1984; Ivanov and Tekerlekov, 1989). Subsequently, a modification of CFT, micro CFT was developed, in which 96 well microtiter plates were used instead of tubes (Darbyshire *et al.,* 1972).

In India, virus type identification by guinea pig cross protection test was replaced by CFT (tube test) in the year 1964-65 (Anon, 1964-65). Subsequently, the micro CFT was adopted for this purpose (Rai, 1980 a and b). Although CFT was a fast method it needed high virus load and results were some times affected by pro-and anti-complementary activities of the test sample (Ferris and Dawson, 1988).

4.2. Virus isolation

Primary cell culture of bovine (Sellers, 1955; Snowden, 1966,; House and House 1989), ovine (Hess *et al.,* 1963; Singh *et al.,* 1969; Nair and Uppal 1983) and porcine (Bachrach *et al.,* 1955) origin have exhibited susceptibility to FMDV from infected tissues. However, the most sensitive culture system for virus isolation is primary bovine thyroid cells (Snowden, 1966) but cryopreservation of bovine thyroid cells directly after trypsinization results in the loss of susceptibility to FMDV (House and House, 1989). Some stable cell lines, like IBRS-2 (Nair, 1987), MVPK-1 clone 7 (Dinka *et al.,* 1977; Nair, 1987), LFBK cell line (Swaney, 1988) and BHK-21 (Swaney 1976; House *et al.,* 1988) are also susceptible to FMDV and so are most desirable for diagnostic system but these are less sensitive than primary cells for detecting low amount of infectivity (Clarke and Spier, 1980).

Revenson and Segura (1963) reported that FMDV grew well on BHK-21 cell line enabling large scale production of antigen with good complement fixing properties. The BHK-21 cell culture provides better growth for FMDV than the suspension culture (Girard, 1975; Clarke and Spier, 1977, 1980).It has also been reported that with subsequent passage in BHK-21 clone 13 cell line, the titre of FMDV increased significantly (Sellers,1955). Nair (1987) reported that the susceptibility and infectivity titers of IBRS-2 and MVPK cell lines were less as compared to BHK-21 cells, and thus had no advantage over BHK-21 cell line for vaccine production. Mishra *et al.,* (1995) also adapted FMDV field isolates to BHK-21 clone 13 cells in 3-7 serial passage.

Goel and Rai (1985) reported that the field isolates of FMDV could be passaged in BHK-21 clone 13 monolayer cell culture, which showed characteristic CPE and were readily adapted between 3rd and 5th passage. The CPE usually develops within 48 hours, if no CPE is detected the cells should be frozen and thawed, used to inoculate fresh cultures and examined for CPE for another 48 hours (OIE, 2009). An alternative to the virus isolation is cell suspension plaque test which also quantify the virus present in sample (Barteling, 1982). However, the cell culture system is laborious, time consuming and relatively low sensitive. It also requires careful handling of specimens and a biosafety laboratory.

4.3. Virus neutralization test (VNT)

With the availability of cell culture techniques and the realization that FMDV can be grown in in-vitro cultured cells made possible the adaption of neutralization test for routine type identification of FMDV isolates and were found to be more specific than CFT (Rweyemamu et al, 1982). Subsequently micro-neutralization test (MNT) was used for the assessment of antigenic variation in field strains, as it correlated well with cattle protection test (Forman, 1975; Rweyemamu, 1984). But it was observed that, minimal heterotypic contamination in the sample could interfere with precise type identification of the virus (Rweyemamu *et al.,* 1978) on the other hand VN test depend on tissue culture and are more prone to variability than ELISA and also require biocontainment facilities.

4.4. Enzyme linked immunosorbent assay (ELISA)

ELISA came into use as diagnostic methods for many infectious diseases around the year 1975 till then it has been used as one of the most accepted serological techniques. The first report of use of an Indirect ELISA to screen cattle for antibodies against FMDV was that of Abu Elzein and Crowther (1978). Subsequently, a sandwich ELISA using convalescent bovine immunoglobulin (Igs) as capture and anti-146S guinea pig sera as tracing sera was found suitable for detection and quantification of FMD virus in infected tissue culture fluid and epithelial tissue samples (Crowther and Abu Elzein, 1979). The use of anti-146S rabbit immunoglobulin in place of convalescent bovine immunoglobulin as capture antibody increased the sensitivity of sandwich ELISA (Ouldridge *et al.,* 1982).

Later ELISA and its various modifications were applied for detection, typing and strain differentiation of FMDV isolates with better sensitivity than CFT and, the results were comparable to that obtained with MNT (Abu Elzein and Crowther, 1978 and 1979; Rai and Lahiri, 1981; Have et al, 1983; Hamblin *et al.,* 1984; Ouldridge *et al.,* 1984; Roeder and Smith, 1987; Pattnaik and Venkataramanan, 1989 a & b). Liquid phase blocking ELISA using bovine convalescent sera for characterization of field isolates was done and result tallied with conventional VNT (Kitching et al, 1988;

Pattnaik *et al.,* 1991; Lunt *et al.,* 1994;). ELISA results were much more reproducible than those obtained with VNT and are not influenced by variations in tissue culture susceptibility. At the FAO/WRL for FMD, the preferred procedure for the detection of FMDV antigen and identification of viral serotypes is ELISA (Paiba *et al.,* 1987; Ferris and Dawson, 1988). The results can be obtained within 3-4 hours after sample is received by the laboratory; a negative sample is confirmed by inoculation of sample into sensitive cultures followed by confirmation of the virus serotype by ELISA.

In India, indirect ELISA was initially used for detection of FMDV antigen in infected cell culture fluid, mice carcass and cattle tongue as well as antibodies in sera samples (Rai and Lahiri, 1981; Pattnaik and Venkataramanan, 1989a). Later a sandwich ELISA was used for subtype analysis of FMDV isolates (Pattnaik. and Venkataramanan, 1989b). Subsequently, a Sandwich ELISA was developed for detection and typing of FMDV directly from field materials (Bhattacharya *et al.,* 1996). Although ELISA is far finer to CFT, a large number of samples failed to give positive results and such negative sample has to be confirmed by inoculation of sample into sensitive cultures (Marvin and Barry, 2004) followed by confirmation of the virus serotype by ELISA taking 4 more days, a time frame compatible with the need to rapidly detect disease and initiate and appropriate disease control strategy. As a consequence, there is a need of an alternative assay system that allows more rapid confirmation of clinical diagnosis with more sensitivity and this has result in development of polymerase chain reaction (PCR) or the more recent real-time PCR.

4.5. Reverse transcription - Polymerase chain reaction (RT-PCR)

Polymerase chain reaction was invented by, Kary Mullis in 1983 (Saiki *et al.,* 1985; Mullis *et al.,* 1987) since then it has been the most widely use nucleic acid based diagnostic techniques. With the development of RT-PCR to amplify RNA targets many workers have assessed the usefulness of it as a reliable tool for FMD diagnosis (Meyer *et al.,*1991; Laor *et al.,*1992; Hofner *et al.,*1993; Rodriguez *et al.,*1994) and in parallel with conventional assays (Marquardt *et al.*,1995; Callens *et al.*,1998 and 1999). A particularly high sensitivity was reported by RT-PCR ELISA (Callens *et al.*, 1998; Alexandersen *et al.*, 2000). A specific RT-PCR was developed and validated for the detection of the polymerase gene (3D) of FMD with an analytical sensitivity of equal to, to 1000 times higher than that of a single passage virus isolation (Moonen, 2003).

In a study to compare the sensitivity of assays for the diagnosis of FMD, a cell suspension plaque test on BHK21-CT cells and a reverse transcription nested PCR (RT-nPCR) were used to examine nasal swabs and probang samples obtained from FMDV infected cattle, it has been observed that examination of nasal swab revealed a higher number of infected animals using RT-nPCR than by the used of the plaque test and for probang samples both test gave approximately equivalent result (Moss & Haas, 1999). PCR products generated have currently only been analyzed by gel electrophoresis exposing to the chance of post PCR contamination. However PCR offers potential advantages over other conventional tests. The risk of false negative associated with poor sample handling is limited. Because virus, if present, would be inactivated by RNA extraction, it would be acceptable to use lower level biosafety. Further, cell culture loses the sensitivity due to presence of inhibitors like interferons and presence of some enzymatic inhibitors. Several studies have compared Reverse Transcription (RT-PCR) methods with FMDV isolation (Donn *et al.*, 1994; Murphy *et al.*, 1994; Callens *et al.*, 1998; Reid *et al.*, 1998, 1999;2000, Moss and Haas, 1999). The sensitivity of the methods reach similar to or greater than virus isolation techniques and these can supplement or go in parallel, but not replace, the routine procedures for diagnosis of FMDV. Detection of all seven serotypes of the virus with each of the serotype specific primers in selected RT-PCR protocols at OIE/FAO World Reference Laboratory for FMD (WRL), Pirbright demonstrated suitable specificity and detected cell culture passage isolate with some success but were not adequate for the serotyping of suspension prepared from clinical samples of epithelium. RT-PCR though has pave the way to more sensitive and rapid test in the field of molecular diagnosis, serotyping of FMDV has been of difficult and this has been solved with the advent of multiplex PCR (mPCR).

4.6. Multiplex Polymerase Chain Reaction (mPCR)

PCR has revolutionized the field of infectious disease diagnosis. To overcome the inherent disadvantage of cost and to improve the diagnostic capacity of the test, multiplex PCR, a variant of the test in which more than one target sequence is amplified using more than one pair of primers, has been developed. This modified technique was originally developed to detect distinct/genetic alterations in large regions of human genome (Chamberlain *et al.,* 1988). Afterwards, mPCR was used for the detection and differentiation of multiple pathogens/different strains of the same pathogen. It has additional advantages such as cost-effectiveness and rapidity. There are reports on the use of mPCR for differential diagnosis of FMDV serotypes (Vangrysperre and Clercq, 1996; Callens and Clercq, 1997). One such PCR (Callens and De Clercq, 1997) was evaluated in WRL FMD Pirbright and found to work on tissue samples with limited success (Reid *et al.,* 1999).To improve the over all diagnostic sensitivity and to provide tools for serotyping FMDV, multiplex PCR arrays have been developed to detect FMDV in infected tissue and food samples (Bao *et al.,* 2008).

The concept of using multiplex PCR to detect FNDV has also been examined by others (Fernandez *et al.,* 2008; Hindson *et al.,* 2008).Multiplex PCR has been applied to the successful differentiation among the SAT serotype, whereas other have utilized this approach to discriminate among O, A, Asia1 and C isolate native to India. An advantage of multiplex PCR systems, compared with probe-based assays, is that the intrinsic design does not rely on a probe for a single conserved gene or region of the genome. Rather, the multiplex system is designed to survey multiple regions of the genome simultaneously, thereby increasing the probability of detection (Elnifro *et al.,* 2000). To date, these mPCR assays are limited to partial serotyping of FMDV because no existing multiplex PCR assay offer complete coverage for all seven serotype (Stanley *et al.,* 2009). Multiplex PCR for differential diagnosis of various vesicular diseases like Vesicular Stomatitis, Swine

Vesicular Disease, Vesicular Exanthema and FMDV have also been described (Nunez *et al.,* 1998; Lomakina *et al.,* 2004). Recently, mPCR for differentiation of Indian FMDV serotypes has been developed and evaluated on tongue epithelium and cell culture samples (Giridharan *et al.,* 2005).

4.7. Real-Time Polymerase Chain Reaction

The use of polymerase chain reaction (PCR) in molecular diagnostics has increased to the point where it is now accepted as the gold standard for detecting nucleic acids from a number of origin and it has become an essential tool in the research laboratory (Mackay *et al.,*2002). The potential of this format to provide sensitive, specific and swift detection and quantification of viral RNAs has made it an indispensible tool for state-of-the-art diagnostics of important human and animal viral pathogens (Hoffmann *et al.,* 2009). Real time PCR has engendered wider acceptance of PCR due to its improved rapidity and sensitivity (Mackay *et al.,* 2002) overcoming poor precision, low sensitivity, low resolution, absence of automation, only size based discrimination, absence of expression of results in numbers, poor quantitative performance (Ethidium bromide for staining is not very quantitative) and post PCR processing, rendering the conventional PCR not very suitable for accurate diagnosis.

There are currently five main chemistries used for the detection of PCR product during real-time PCR. These are the DNA binding fluorophores, the 5′ endonuclease, adjacent linear and hairpin oligoprobes and the self-fluorescing amplicons (Mackay *et al.,* 2002). This approach is a highly sensitive technique enabling simultaneous amplification and quantification of specific nucleic acid sequences. In addition to enhanced sensitivity, the benefits of real-time PCR assays over conventional endpoint detection methods include their large dynamic range, a reduced risk of cross contamination, an ability to be scaled up for high throughput applications and the potential for accurate target quantification (Nazarenko *et al.,* 1997; Schweiger *et al.,* 2000; Black *et al.,* 2002) Real-time PCR assays recommended by the World Organization for animal health (OIE) for detection of FMDV incorporate universal primers and fluorescent-labeled probes that recognized conserved region within the 5′ UTR (Reid *et al.,* 2002) or conserved gene regions within the RNA-dependent RNA polymerase gene (3Dpol) (Callahan *et al.,* 2002).The use of a specific probe facilitates an increase in specificity compared to conventional agarose-gel-based PCR assays (Bustin, 2000; Bustin *et al.,* 2005).

Recently, TaqMan technology has combined the 5′nuclease activity of the Taq DNA polymerase and forster resonance energy transfer to detect and quantify amplification product in a closed tube format. Using this technology Real-Time PCR has been developed to detect the nucleic acid (Livak *et al.,* 1995; Morris *et al.,* 1996; Kessler *et al.,* 2000). This is most sensitive and rapid method to detect the nucleic acid. The viral RNA can be consistently detected over a seven log range, the lowest of which corresponded to as few as 10-100 RNA per volume tested. The test can be performed in 2 hour or less on a portable instrument and sample can be held at ambient temperatures. Real Time chemistry allows for the detection of PCR amplification during the early phases of the reaction and as the name suggest, real time PCR monitor the progress of a PCR reaction in the real time. At the same time, a relatively small amount of PCR product (DNA, CDNA or RNA) can be quantified. Measuring the kinetics of the reaction in the early phases of PCR provides a distinct advantage over traditional PCR detection. Traditional methods use agarose gels for detection of PCR amplification at the final phase or end point of the PCR reaction which is associated with considerable hands on time, posses a serious hazard for amplification product carryover, and limits the number of specimen that can be processed simultaneously. It is hard to differentiate the 5 fold changes on gel whereas Real Time PCR is able to detect even two fold changes (e.g.10 vs. 20 copies). In addition to the widely exploited 5′- nuclease (TaqMan) system using dual-labelled probes (Reid *et al.,* 2002; Callahan *et al.,* 2002; Oem *et al.,* 2005) and modified MGB probes (Moniwa *et al.,*2007), assays have also been developed using other rRT-PCR formats such as those using hybridization probes (Moonen *et al.,* 2003) and PriProET (Rasmussen *et al.,* 2003).

The greatest problem facing the diagnostic application of PCR is the production of false positive results. They are attributable to contamination by nucleic acids, particularly from the previously amplified material (carry over). Any contaminant, even the smallest airborne remnant carried over from the previous PCR procedure or from a strongly positive sample (contamination), may be multiplied and produce a false positive results. In the Real time PCR, the problem of carry-over is significantly reduced because of the real time measuring principle, which is based on closed tube system. In order to increase assay throughput and minimise operator errors, Real-Time PCR assays for FMDV has also be automated using robots for nucleic acid extraction and liquid handling equipment to set-up the reaction mixes (Reid *et al.,* 2003; Moonen *et al.,* 2003). The assay has also been applied for FMDV and it is capable of detecting all seven serotypes (Reid *et al.,* 2001, 2002, 2003, Oleksiewicz *et al.,* 2001; Alexandersen *et al.,* 2001, 2002,2003; Callhan *et al.,* 2002; Zhang and Alexandersen, 2003; Barnett et al. 2004; Cox *et al.,* 2005). First inter-assay/laboratory equivalence investigation (Ferris *et al.,*2006), participated by five European reference laboratories for detection of FMDV has observed that the best of the Real-Time PCR assays used in each laboratory gave comparable results unlike the VI results which were highly variable. Performance of three real time instrument the LightCycler.2 (Roche), the SmartCycler I I (Cepheid), and the SDS 7900HT (AB) was compared for detection of FMDV and has successfully identified the FMDV genome and beta actin mRNA from several sources of infected nasal and oral swabs, as well as probang samples (Moniwa *et al.,*2007). In addition to extensive testing of vesicular epithelium samples, the performance of rRT-PCR has recently been assessed on milk (Reid *et al.,* 2006) and ==probang" samples (Sammin *et al.,* 2007). Automated real-time RT-PCR has been compared with VI and antigen-detection ELISA with result showing more positive by real time PCR indicating that the real-time PCR has higher sensitivity than VI for the detection of FMDV in epithelial samples (Shaw *et al.,* 2004).

The development of multi-colour real-time PCR cyclers and ==ready-to-use" commercial multiplex real-time PCR kits has also made it possible to combine several assays within a single tube. Major advantages of multiplexing include a reduced sample requirement, which is especially important when sample material is scarce (Persson *et al.,* 2005; Belak, 2007), and the ability to combine assays with an internal control system (Hoffmann *et al.,* 2006). However, it is important to optimize these assays in order to limit competitive interactions that may significantly impact upon assay sensitivity. The combined properties of high sensitivity and specificity, low contamination risk, and speed has made real-time PCR technology a highly attractive alternative to tissue culture- or immunoassay-based methods for diagnosing many infectious diseases (Espy *et al.,* 2006). Clinical diagnostic applications and the use of real-time PCRs are growing exponentially, and real-time PCR is rapidly replacing conventional PCR and other established diagnostic methods such as antigen-ELISA and cell culture isolation.

References

Abu Elzein, E.M.E. and Crowther, J.R. (1978). Enzyme-labelled immunosorbent assay techniques in foot-and-mouth disease virus research. J. Hyg. Camb., 80: 391-399.

Abu Elzein, E.M.E. and Crowther, J.R. (1979). The specific detection of foot and mouth disease virus whole particle (146S) by Enzyme labelled immunosorbent assay. J. Hyg. Camb., 83: 127 -134.

Acharya, R.; Fry, E.; Stuart, D.; Fox, G.; Rowlands, D. and Brown, F. (1989). The three-Dimensional structure of foot-and-mouth disease virus at 2.9 A° resolution. Nature, 337: 709-716.

Ahuja, K.L.; Kumar, A. and Prasad, S. (1996). Incidence and distribution of foot-and-mouth disease virus types in North-West India (1991-93). Indian J. Virol., 12: 125-127.

Ahuja, K.L.; Kumar, A.; Prasad, S. and Sharma, R. (1986). Incidence and distribution of foot-and-mouth disease virus types in North-West India (1982-84). Indian J. Anim. Sci., 56: 503-505.

Alexandersen, S.; Zhang, Z. and Donaldson, A.I. (2002). Aspects of the persistence of foot-and-mouth disease virus in animals - the carrier problem. Microbes and Infection., 4: 1099-1110

Alexandersen, S.; Forsyth, M.A.; Reid, S.M. and Belsham, G.J. (2000). Development of reverse transcription-PCR (oligonucleotide probing) enzyme-linked immunosorbent assays for diagnosis and preliminary typing of foot-and-mouth disease: a new system using simple and aqueous-phase hybridization. J. Clin. Microbiol., 38: 4604–4613.

Alexandersen, S.; Olesksiewicz, M.B. and Donaldson, A.I. (2001). The early pathogenesis of foot-and-mouth disease in pig infected by contact: A quantitative time-course study using Taq Man RT-PCR. J. Gen. Virol., 82: 747 – 755.

Alexandersen, S.; Zhang Z.; Donaldson, A.I. and Garland, A.J. (2003). Pathogenesis and diagnosis of foot-and-mouth disease . J. Comp. Pathol., 129 (1): 1-36.

Amaral-Doel, C.M.F.; Owen, N.E.; Ferris, N.P.; Kitching, R.P. and Doel, T.R. (1993). Detection foot-and-mouth disease viral sequences in clinical specimens and ethyleneimine-inactivated preparations by the polymerase chain reaction. Vaccine, 11: 415-421.

Anonymous (1964-1965). Annual report of the Indian veterinary research institute, Mukteswar

Anonymous (1991). Report, Institute of Rural Management, Anand.

Bachrach, H.L. (1968). Foot-and-mouth disease virus. Annu. Rev. Microbiol., 22: 201-244.

Bachrach, H.L.; Hess, W.R. and Callis, J.J. (1955). Foot-and-mouth disease virus: its growth and cytopathogenicity in tissue culture. Science, 122: 1269-1270.

Bao, H.F.; Li, D.; Guo, J.H.; Lu, Z.J.; Chen, Y.L.; Liu, Z.X.; Liu, X.T.and Xie, Q.G., (2008). A highly sensitive and specific multiplex RT- PCR to detect foot-and-mouth disease virus in tissue and foot samples. Arch. Virol., 153:205-209.

Barman, N.N.; Sarma, D.K.; Das, S. and Patgiri, G.P. (1999). Foot- and mouth disease in wild and semi-domesticated animals of the North Eastern states of India. Indian J. Anim. Sci., 69 (10): 781-783.

Barnett, P.V.; Keel, P.; Reid, S.; Armstrong, R.M.; Statham, R.J.; Voyce, C.; Aggarwal, N. and Cox, S.J. (2004). Evidence that high potency foot-and-mouth disease vaccine inhibits local virus replication and prevents the "carrier" state in sheep. Vaccine, 22: 1221-32.

Barteling, S.J., Wagenaar, F. and Gielkens, A.L. (1982). The positively charged structural virus protein (VP1) of foot-and-mouth disease virus (type

O1) contains a highly basic part which may be involved in early virus-cell interaction. J Gen Virol., 62: 357-61.

Bedson, S.P.; Maitland, H.B.and Burbury, Y.M., (1927). 2nd Report, Foot-and-Mouth Disease Research Committee, HMSO, London. p.99. (cited by Brown, F.2003. Virus Res., 91: 3-7).

Belak, S. (2007). Molecular diagnosis of viral diseases, present trends and future aspects. A view from the OIE Collaborating Centre for the Application of Polymerase Chain Reaction Methods for Diagnosis of Viral Diseases in Veterinary Medicine. Vaccine., 25: 5444– 5452.

Belnap, D.M.; McDermott, B.M.; Filman, Jr. D.J.; Cheng, N.; Trus, B.L.; Zuccola, H.J.; Racaniello, V.R.; Hogle, J.M. and Steven, A.C. (2000). Three dimensional structure of poliovirus receptor bound to poliovirus. Proc. Natl. Acad. Sci. USA., 97: 73-78.

Belsham, G.J. (1993). Distinctive features of foot-and-mouth disease virus, a member of the picornavirus family; aspects of virus protein synthesis, protein processing and structure. Prog. Biophys. Mol. Biol., 60: 41-60.

Belsham, G.J.; Abrams, C.C.; King, A.M.; Roosien, J. and Vlak, J.M. (1991). Myristoylation of foot-and-mouth disease virus capsid protein precursors is independent of other viral proteins and occurs in both mammalian and insect cells. J. Gen. Virol., 72: 747-751

Bhattacharya, S.; Pattnaik, B. and Venkataramanan, R. (1996). Development and application of sandwich enzyme linked immunosorbent assay (ELISA) for type identification of foot-and-mouth disease (FMD) virus in direct field materials. Indian. J. Anim. Sci., 66: 1201-1209.

Bittle, J.L.; Houghten, R.A.; Alexxander, H.; Shinnick, T.M.; Sutcliffe, J.G; Learner, R.A.; Rowlands, D.J. and Brown, F. (1982) protection against foot-and-mouth disease by immunization with a chemically synthesized peptide predicted from the viral nucleotide sequence. Nature, 298: 30-33.

Black, E.M.; Lowings, J.P.; Smith, J.; Heaton, P.R.; McElhinney, L.M. (2002). A rapid RT-PCR method to differentiate six established genotypes of rabies and rabies-related viruses using TaqMan technology. J. Virol. Methods., 105 (1): 25-35.

Brooksby, J.B. (1982). Portraits of viruses: foot-and-mouth disease virus. Intervirology., 18: 1-10.

Brooksyby, J.B. and Rogers, J. (1957). Methods used in typing the virus of foot-and- mouth disease at Pirbright, 1950-55. In method of typing and cultivation of foot and mouth disease virus .project no 208. Paris, OEEC. 1957: 31-34.

Bruner, D.W and Gillespie, J.H. (1973). The family Picornaviridae. In: Hagan's Infectious disease of domestic animals, 6th Edn. pp. 1207-1208.

Bunch, T.; Rieder, E. and Mason, P. (1994). Sequence of the S fragment of foot-and mouth disease virus type A12. Virus Genes., 8: 173-175.

Burrows, R; Mann, J.A.; Garland, A.J.; Greig, A. and Goodridge, D. (1981). The pathogenesis of natural and simulated natural foot-and-mouth-disease infection in cattle. J. Comp. Pathol., 91: 599-609.

Bustin, S.A. (2000). Absolute quantification of mRNA using real-time reverse transcription polymerase chain reaction assays. J. Mol. Endocrinol., 25 (2): 169–193.

Bustin, S.A.; Benes, V.; Nolan, T. and Pfaffl, M.W. (2005). Quantitative real-time RT-PCR—a perspective. J. Mol. Endocrinol., 34 (3): 597–601.

Buxton, A. and Fraser, G. (1977). Animal Microbiology., Vol. 2. Blackwell Scientific Publication, Oxford.

Callahan, J.D.; Brown, F.; Osorio, F.A.; Sur, J.H.; Kramer, E.; Long, G.W.; Lubroth, J.; Ellis, S.J.; Shoulars, K.S.; Gaffney, K.L.; Rock, D.L. and Nelson, W.M. (2002). Use of a portable real-time reverse transcriptase-polymerase chain reaction assay for rapid detection of foot-and-mouth disease virus. J. Am. Vet. Med. Assoc., 220 (11): 1636–1642.

Callens, M. and De Clercq, K. (1997). Differentiation of the seven serotypes of foot-and-mouth disease virus by reverse transcriptase chain reaction. J. Virol. Methods., 67: 35-44.

Callens, M. and De Clercq, K. (1999). Highly sensitive detection of swine vesicular disease virus based on a single tube RT-PCR system and DIG-ELISA detection. J. Virol. Methods., 77: 87-99.

Callens, M.; De Clercq, K.; Gruia, M. and Danes, M. (1998). Detection of footand- mouth disease by reverse transcription polymerase chain reaction and virus isolation in contact sheep without clinical signs of foot-and-mouth disease. Vet. Q., 20: 37–40.

Capozzo, A.V.; Burke, D.J.; Fox, J.W.; Bergmann, I.E.; La, Torre, J.L. and Grigera P.R. (2002). Expression of foot and mouth disease virus non-structural polypeptide 3ABC induces histone H3 cleavage in BHK21 cells. Virus Res., 90, 91-96.

Cavanagh, D.; Sangar, D.V.; Rowlands, D.J. and Brown, F. (1977). Immunogenic and cell attachment sites of foot-and-mouth disease virus: further evidence for their location in a single capsid polypeptide, J. Gen. Virol., 35: 149-158.

Clarke, J.B and Spier, R.E. (1977). Studies on susceptibility to foot-and-mouth disease virus of BHK cell cultures derived from various sources. Int. Symp. FMD, Lyon, 1976. Develop. Biol. Stand., 35: 61-66.

Clarke, J.B. and Spier, R.E. (1980). Variation in the susceptibility of BHK populations and cloned cell lines to three strains of foot-and-mouth disease virus. Arch. Virol., 63: 1-9.

Costa-Goami, M.P.; Bergmann, I.E.; Scodeller, E.A.; Auge, de, Mello, P.; Gomez, I. and La, Torre, J.L. (1984). Heterogeneity of the polyribocytidylic acid tract in aphthovirus: biochemical and biological studies of viruses carrying polyribocytidylic acid tractsof different lengths. J. Virol., 51: 799-805.

Cox, S.J.; Voyce C.; Parida, S.; Reid, S. M.; Hamblin, P.A.; Paton, D.J. and Barnett, P.V. (2005). Protection against direct-contact challenge following emergency FMD vaccination of cattle and the effect on virus excretion from the oropharynx. Vaccine., 23: 1106-13.

Crowther, J.R. and Abu, Elzein, E.M.E. (1979). Application of the enzyme linked immunosorbent assays to the detection and identification of foot-and-mouth disease virus. J.Hyg.Camb., 83:513-519.

Darbyshire, J.H.; Hedger, R.S. and Arrowsmith, A.E.M. (1972). Comparative complement fixation studies with subtypes strains of foot-and-mouth disease virus. J. Hyg. Camb., 70:171-180

Dinka, S.K.; Swaney, L.M. and Mc Vicar, J.W. (1977). Selection of a stable clone of the MVPK-1 foetal porcine kidney cell line for assays of foot-and-mouth disease virus. Can. J. Microbiol., 23: 295-299.

Domingo, E., Escarmís, C., Martínez, M. A., Martínez-Salas, E. and Mateu, M. G. (1992) Foot-andmouth disease virus populations are quasispecies, Curr. Topics Microbiol. Immunol. 176, 33-47.

Domingo, E.; Mateu, M. G.; Martínez, M. A.; Dopazo, J.; Moya, A. and Sobrino, F. (1990). Genetic variability and antigenic diversity of foot-and-mouth disease virus. In : Applied Virology Research. Kurstak, E., Marusk, R.G., Murphy, S.A .and Van Regenmortel, M. H. V. (eds.), 2: 233-266.

Donaldson, A.I; Gibson, C.F.; Oliver, R.; Hamlin, C. and Kitching, R.F. (1987). Infection of cattle by airborne foot-and-mouth disease virus: minimal doses with O2 and SAT2 strains. Res. Vet. Sci., 43: 339–346.

Donnelly, M.L.; Gani, D.; Flint, M.; Monaghan, S. and Ryan, M.D. (1997). The cleavage activities of aphthovirus and cardiovirus 2A proteins. J. Gen. Virol., 78: 13-21.

Dorsch-Hasler, K.; Yogo, Y. and Wimmer, E. (1975). Replication of picornaviruses. I. Evidence from in vitro RNA synthesis that poly (A) of the poliovirus genome is genetically coded. J. Virol., 16: 1512-1517.

Dutta, P.K.; Mahanta, P.N. and Chakraborty, A.K. (1979). FMD in Mithun. Vet Rec., 113:114.

Dutta, P.K.; Sharma, G. and Das, S.K. (1984). Occurrence of foot-and-mouth disease and distribution of virus type in the hill states of North Eastern region of India. Indian J. Anim. Sci., 4: 117-118.

Elnifro, E.M.; Ashshi, A.M.; Cooper, R.J. and Klapper, P.F. (2000). Multiplex PCR: optimization and application in diagnostic virology. Clin. Microbiol. Rev., 13: 559-550.

Espy, M.J.; Uhl, J.R.; Sloan, L.M.; Buckwalter, S.P.; Jones, M.F.; Vetter, E.A.; Yao, J.D.; Wengenack, N.L.; Rosenblatt, J.E.; Cockerill 3rd F.R. and Smith, T.F. (2006). Real-time PCR in clinical microbiology: applications for routine laboratory testing. Clin. Microbiol. Rev., 19: 165–256.

Ferguson, N.M.; Donelly, C.A. and Anderson. R.M. (2001). The foot-and-mouth epidemic in Great Britain: pattern of spread and impact of interventions. Science., 292: 1155–1160.

Fernandez, J.; Aguero, M.; Romero, L.; Sanchez, C.; Belak, S.; Arras, M. and Sanchez, Vizcaino, J.M. (2008). Rapid and differential diagnosis of foot-and-mouth disease, swine vesicular disease, and vesicular stomatitis by a new multiplex RT-PCR assay. J. Virol. Methods, 147, 301-311.

Ferris, N.P. and Dawson, M. (1988). Routine application of enzyme-linked immunosorbent assay in comparison with complement fixation for the diagnosis of foot-and-mouth and swine vesicular diseases. Vet. Microbiol., 16, 201–209.

Ferris, N.P.; Donaldson, A.I.; Barnett, I.T.R. and Osborne, R.W. (1984). Inactivation, purification and stability of 146S antigens of foot-and-mouth disease virus for use as reagent in the complement fixation test. Rev. Sci. Tech. O.I.E., 3: 339-350.

Ferris, N.P.; King, D.P.; Reid, S.M.; Hutchings, G.H.; Shaw, A.E.; Paton, D.J.,; Goris, N.; Haas, B.; Hoffmann, B.; Brocchi, E.; Bugnetti, M.; Dekker, A. and De Clercq, K. (2006). Foot-and-mouth disease virus: a first interlaboratory comparison trial to evaluate virus isolation and RT-PCR detection methods. Vet. Microbiol., 117 (2–4): 130–140.

Forman, A.J. (1975). A comparison of some immunological methods for the differentiation of strains of FMD virus. J. Hyg. Camb., 74, 215-225.

Fracastorius, H. (1546). De contagion et contagiosus morbis et curatione, Book 1. Chapter 12, Venecia (cited by Sobrino *et al.,* 2001)

Fred Brown. (2003). The history of research in foot-and-mouth disease Virus Research., 91, 3-7

Girard, H.C. (1975). Evolution of BHK cells. Rept. Mtg. FAO, Brescia, Italy : 20-23

Giridharan, P.; Hemadri, D.; Tosh , C.; Sanyal, A. and Bandhopadhyay, S.K. (2005). Development and evaluation of multiplex PCR for differentiation of foot-and mouth disease virus strains native to India. J. Virol. Methods., 125: 1-11.

Goel, A.C. and Rai, A. (1985).Growth curve, plaque assay and inactivation studies of FMD virus subtypes O5, O1 and O6 of Indian origin. Indian J. Comp. Microbiol. Immunol. Infect. Dis., 6 (1): 16-28.

Grubman, M.J. and Baxt, B. (2004). Foot -and-mouth disease. Clin. Microbiol. Rev., 17: 465-93.

Hambling, C.; Armstrong, R.M. and Hedger, R.S. (1984). Rapid enzyme linked immunosorbent assay for the detection of foot-and –mouth disease in epithelial tissues. Vet. Microbiol., 9: 435-443.

Harris, T.J. and Brown, F. (1977). Biochemical analysis of a virulent and an avirulent strain of foot-and-mouth disease virus. J. Gen. Virol., 34: 87-105.

Have, P.; Lei, J.C. and Schjerning-Thiesen, K. (1983). An engyme linked immunosorbent assay (ELISA) for the primary diagnosis of foot-and-mouth disease: characterization and comparison with complement fixation. Rpt. Sess. Res. Gp. Stand. Tech. Comm. Eur. Comm. Control of FMD (FAO), Lelystad. pp 34-42.

Herold, J. and Andino, R. (2001). Poliovirus RNA replication requires genome circularization through a protein-protein bridge. Mol. Cell., 7: 581-591.

Hindson, B.J.; Reid, S.M.; Baker, B.R.; Ebert, K.; Ferris, N.P.; Tammero, L.F.; Lenhoff, R.J.; Naraghi-Arani, P.; Vitalis, E.A.; Slezak, T.R.; Hullinger, P.J. and King, D.P. (2008). Diagnostic evaluation of multiplexed reverse transcription-PCR microsphere array assay for detection of foot-and-mouth and look-alike disease viruses. J. Clin. Microbiol., 46: 1081-1089.

Hoffmann, B.; Martin, B.; Reid, S.M.; Peter, M.; Oura, C.A.L.; Piet, A.; van Rijn Slomka, M.J.; Jill Bank Ian H.; Brown , D. J.; Alexander Donald, P. and King, A.M. (2009). A review of RT-PCR technologies used in veterinary virology and disease control: Sensitive and specific diagnosis of five livestock diseases notifiable to the World Organisation for Animal Health. Veterinary Microbiology, 139: 1–23.

Hofner, M.C.; Carpenter, W.C. and Donaldson, A.I. (1993). Detection of foot-and-mouth disease virus RNA in clinical samples and cell culture isolates by amplication of capsid coding region. J. Virol. Methods, 42: 53-6

House, C. and House, J.A. (1989). Evaluation of Techniques to Demonstrate Foot-and-mouth Disease Virus in Bovine Tongue Epithelium: Comparison of the Sensitivity of Cattle, Mice, Primary Cell Cultures, Cryopreserved Cell Cultures and Established Cell Lines. Vet. Microbiol., 20: 99-109.

House, J.A.; House, C. and Llewellyn, M.E. (1988). Characteristics of the porcine kidney cell line IB-RS-2 clone D10 (IR-RS-2 D10) which is free of hog cholera virus. Can. J. Comp. Med., 24: 677-682.

Ivanov, Y.A. and Tekerlekov, P. (1989). Typing Aphthovirus by the micro-complement fixation test. Veterinarya Sbrikà., 87: 18-21.

Jackson, T.; King, A.M.; Stuart, D.I. and Fry, E. (2003). Structure and receptor binding. Virus Res., 91: 33-46.

Jackson, T.; Mould, A.P.; Sheppard, D. and King, A.M. (2002). Integrin vß1 is a receptor for foot-and-mouth disease virus. J. Virol., 76: 935-941.

Jang, S.K.; Krausslich, H.G.; Nicklin, M.J.; Duke, G.M.; Palmenberg, A.C. and Wimmer, E. (1988). A segment of the 5' nontranslated region of encephalomyocarditis virus RNA directs internal entry of ribosomes during\ in vitro translation. J. Virol., 62: 2636-2643.

Kessler, H.H.; Muhlbauer, G.; Rinner, B.; Stelzl, .E.; Berger, A.; Dorr, H.W.; Santner, B.; Marth, E. and Rabenau, H. (2000). Detection of Herpes Simplex virus DNA by real-time PCR. J. Clin. Microbiol., 38: 2638-42.

Kitching, R.P.; Rendle, R. and Ferris, N.P. (1988). Rapid correlation between field isolates and vaccine strains of FMD virus. Vaccine., 6: 403-408.

Knowles, N.J.; Samuel, A.R.; Davies, P.R.; Kitching, R.P. and Donaldson, A.I. (2001). Outbreak of foot-and-mouth disease virus serotype O in the UK caused by a pandemic strain. Vet. Rec., 148: 258–259.

Kumar, A.; Prasad. S.; Ahuja, K.L.; Tewari, S.C.; Dogra, S.C. and Garg, D.N. (1983). Distribution pattern of foot-and-mouth disease virus types in North-West India (1979-81). Haryana Veterinarian, 22: 28-30.

Laor, O.; Torgersen, H.; Yadin, H. and Becker, Y. (1992). Detection of FMDV RNA amplified by the polymerase chain reaction (PCR). J. Virol. Methods., 36: 197-208.

Laporte, J. and Lenoir, G. (1973) Structural proteins of foot-and-mouth disease virus, J. Gen. Virol., 20: 161-168.

Lea, S.; Hernandez, J.; Blakemoore, W.; Brocchi, E.; Curry, S.; Domingo, E.; Fry, E.; Abu-ghazaleh, R.; King, A.; Newman, J.; Stuart, D. and Mateu, M.G. (1994). The structure and antigenicity of a type C foot and mouth disease virus. Structure., 2: 123–139.

Lee, W.M.; Monroe, S.S. and Rueckert, R.R. (1993). Role of maturation cleavage in infectivity of picornaviruses: activation of an infectosome. J. Virol., 67, 2110-2122.

Loeffler, F. and Frosch, P. (1897). Summarischer Bericht uber die Ergebnisse der Untersuchungen zur Erforschung der Maul- und Klauenseuche. Zentbl. Bakteriol. Parasitenkd Abt. I 22: 257–259. (Cited by Marvin and Barry, 2004).

Loeffler, F. and Frosch, P. (1898) Berichte der Kommission zur Erforschung der Maul- und Klauenseuche bei dem Institut für Infectrions-krankheiten in Berlin, Zbl. Bakter Abt. I. Orig., 23: 371-391

Logan, D.; Abu-Ghazaleh, R.; Blakemore, W.; Curry, S.; Jackson, T.; King, A.; Lea, S.; Lewis, R.; Newman, J.; Stuart, D. and Fry, E. (1993). Structure of a major immunogenic site on foot-and mouth disease virus. Nature., 362: 566–568

Lomakina, N.F.; Fallacara, F.; Pacciarini, M.; Amadori, M.; Lomakin, A.I.; Timina, A.M.; Shcherbakova, L.O. and Drygin, V.V. (2004). Application of universal

primers for identification of foot-and-mouth disease virus and swine vesicular disease virus by PCR and PCR ELISA. Arch. Virol., 49: 1155-1170.

Lopez de Quinto, Saiz S. M.; de la Morena, D.; Sobrino, F. and Martinez-Salas, E. (2002). IRES-driven translation is stimulated separately by the FMDV 3'-NCR and poly (A) sequences. Nuc. Acids Res., 30: 4398-4405.

Lunt, R.A.; Linchongsubongkoch, W. and Gleeson, L.J. (1994). A modified liquid phase (LP) blocking ELISA used to assess type O foot-and-mouth disease virus antigenic variation in Thailand. Vet. Microbiol., 42: 79-90.

Mackay, I.M.; Katherine, E.; Arden and Andreas Nitsche. (2002). Survey and Summary Real-time PCR in virology. Nucleic Acids Research., 30: 1292-1305.

Marquardt, O.; Straub, O.C.; Ahl, R. and Hass, B. (1995). Detection of foot-and-mouth disease virus in nasal swabs of asymptomatic cattle by RT-PCR within 24 hours. J. Virol. Methods., 53: 255-261.

Marvin, J.G. and Barry, B. (2004). Foot and Mouth Disease, Clinical Microbiology Review., 17 (2): 465–493.

Mason, P.W.; Bezborodova, S.V. and Henry, T.M. (2002). Identification and characterization of a cis-acting replication element (cre) adjacent to the internal ribosome entry site of foot-and-mouth disease virus. J. Virol., 76: 9686-9694.

Mateu, M. G. (1995). Antibody recognition of picornaviruses and escape from neutralization: a structural view. Virus Res., 38: 1–24.

Meyer, R.F.; Brown, C.C.; House, C.; House, J.A. and Molitor, T.W. (1991). Rapid and sensitive detection of foot-and-mouth disease virus in tissues by enzymatic RNA amplification of the polymerase gene. J. Virol. Methods, 34: 161–172.

Mishra, N.; Mishra, S. and Bhagwan, P.S.K. (1998). Vaccines for small ruminants- Need and development strategies. Livestock International, 2 (8): 9-11.

Mishra, N.; Rai, D.V. and Pattnaik, B. (1995). Strain differentiation of foot-and-mouth disease virus type =Asia1'. Indian J. Anim. Sci., 65: 368-375.

Moniwa, M.; Clavijo, A.; Li,M.; Collignon, B. and Kitching, R.P. (2007). Performance of a foot-and-mouth disease virus reverse transcription polymerase chain reaction with amplification controls between three real-time instruments. J. Vet. Diagn Invest., 19: 9-20.

Moonen, P.; Jan Boonstra.; Renate Hakze-van der Honing.; Christine Boonstra-Leendertse Liesbeth Jacobs. and Aldo, D. (2003). Validation of a Light Cycler–based reverse transcriptase polymerase chain reaction for the detection of foot-and-mouth disease virus. J. Virol. Methods, 113: 35-41.

Morrel, D.J.; Mellur, E.J.C.; Rowlands, D.J. and Brown, F. (1987). Surface structure and RNA-protein interactions of foot-and-mouth disease virus. J. Gen. Virol., 68: 1649-1658.

Morris, T.; Robertson, B. and Gallagher, M. (1996). Rapid reverse transcription- PCR detection of hepatitis C virus RNA in serum by using the TaqMan fluorogenic detection system. J. Clin. Microbiol., 34: 2933-2936.

Moss, A. and Haas, B. (1999). Comparison of the plaque test and reverse transcription nested PCR for the detection of FMDV in nasal swabs and probing samples. J. Virol. Methods, 80: 59–67 .

Mukhopadhyay, A.K. (1992). Distribution of FMD virus types and subtypes in India. Summer Institute on Recent Advances in Diagnosis and Control of FMD, I.V.R.I., Bangalore.

Mullis, K.B.and Faloona, F.A.(1987). Specific synthesis of DNA in vitro via a polymerase-catalyzed reaction. Methods Enzymol., 155: 335-350.

Murphy, F.A.; Gibbs, E.P.J.; Horzinek, M.C. and Studdert, M.J. (1999) Picornaviridae. Veterinary Virology., third edition, Academic Press, London, pp 517-528.

Nair, S.P. (1987). Studies on the susceptibility and growth pattern of foot-and-mouth disease virus vaccine strains in two pig kidney cell lines. Indian J. Comp. Microbiol. Immunol. Infect. Dis., 8 (2):76-81.

Nazarenko, I.A.; Bhatnagar, S.K. and Hohman, R.J. (1997). A closed tube format for amplification and detection of DNA based on energy transfer. Nucleic Acids Res., 25: 2516–2521.

Newman, J.F; Piatti, P.G.; Ryan, M.D. and Brown, F. (1994). Function of minor polypeptides in foot-and-mouth disease virus and poliovirus. Trends. Microbiol., 2: 494-497.

Nishiura H and Omori R. (2010). An Epidemiological Analysis of the Foot-and-Mouth Disease Epidemic in Miyazaki, Japan, .Transboundary and Emerging Diseases in press(doi:10.1111/j.1865-1682.2010.01162)

Nunez, J.; Blanco, E.; Hernandez, T.; Gomez-Tejedor, C.; Martin, M.; Dopazo, J. and Sobrino, F.(1998). A RT-PCR assay for the differential diagnosis of vesicular disease of swine. J. Virol. Methods, 72: 227-235.

Oem, J.K.; Kye S.J.; Lee, K.N.; Park, J.H.; Kim, Y.J.; Song, H.J. and Yeh, M. (2005). Development of synthetic peptide ELISA based on nonstructural protein 2C of foot and mouth disease virus. J. Vet. Sci., 317-25.

Office Of International des Epizooties, OIE (2008a). OIE Terrestrial Manual 2008. Foot and mouth disease. Chapter 2.1.5. pp: 190-217.

Office Of International des Epizooties, OIE (2008b). OIE Terrestrial Manual 2008. Principle of validation of diagnostic assays for infectious disease. Chapter 1.1.4. pp: 190-217

Office Of International des Epizooties, OIE (2009). OIE Terrestrial Manual 2009. Foot and mouth disease. Chapter 2.1.5. pp: 1-29.

Oleksiewicz, M.B.; Donaldson, A.I. and Alexandersen, S. (2001). Development of a novel real-time RT-PCR assay for quantitation of foot-and-mouth disease virus in diverse porcine tissues. J. Virol. Methods, 102: 23–35.

Ouldridge, E.J.; Barnett, P. and Rweyemamu, M.M. (1982). The relative efficiency of two ELISA techniques for the tritration of FMD antigen. Curr. Top. Vet. Med. Anim. Sci., 22: 142-151.

Ouldridge, E.J.; Barnett, P.V.; Hingley, P. J.; Head, M. and Rweyemamu, M.M. (1984). The differentiation of foot-and-mouth disease virus strains using an indirect sandwich enzyme-linked immunosorbent assay saturation model. J. Biol. Stand., 12: 367-377.

Paiba, G.A.; Anderson, J.; Paton, D.J.; Soldan, A.W.; Alexandersen, S.; Corteyn, M.; Wilsden, G.; Hamblin, P.; MacKay, D.K. and Donaldson, A.I. (1987).

Pattnaik, B. and Venkataramanan, R. (1989a). Indirect enzyme linked immunosorbent assay for the detection of FMDV antigen. Indian J. Anim. Sci., 59: 317-322.

Pattnaik, B. and Venkataramanan, R. (1989b). A sandwich enzyme linked immunosorbent assay for subtype analysis of foot-and-mouth disease virus isolate. Indian J. Anim. Sci., 59: 1363-1368.

Pattnaik, B.; Rai, D.V.and Venkataramanan, R.(1991). Specificity of foot-and-mouth disease virus antigen and antibody reaction in liquid phase ELISA. Indian J. Anim. Sci., 61: 235-240.

Pereira, H.G. (1977). Subtyping of foot-and-mouth disease virus. Dev. Biol. Stand., 35: 167-174.

Persson, K.; Hamby, K. and Ugozzoli, L.A. (2005). Four-color multiplex reverse transcription polymerase chain reaction—overcoming its limitations. Anal. Biochem., 344: 33–42.

Pilipenko, E.V.; Gmyl, A.P.; Maslova, S.V.; Svitkin, Y.V.; Sinyakov, A.N. and Agol, V.I. (1992). Prokaryotic-like cis elements in the cap-independent internal initiation of translation on picornavirus RNA. Cell., 68: 119-131.

Pilipenko, E.V.; Poperechny, K.V.; Maslova, S.V.; Melchers, W.J.; Slot, H.J. and Agog, V.I. (1996). Cis-element, oriR, involved in the initiation of (–) strand Poliovirus RNA: a quasi-globular multi-domain RNA structure maintained by tertiary ('kissing') interactions. EMBO J., 15: 5428-5436.

Prasad, S. (1971). Distribution of different types of foot-and-mouth disease virus in North-West region of India. Haryana Veterinarian, 10: 26-29.

Prasad, S.; Goel, M.C.; Sharma, V.K.; Tewari, S.C.; Dogra, S.C.; Pandey, R. and Ramakant. (1978). A note on the incidence and distribution of foot-and-mouth

disease virus types in North-West region of India. Indian J. Anim. Sci., 48: 627-29.

Pyakural, S.; Singh, U. and Singh, N.B. (1976). An outbreak of foot-and-mouth disease in Indian elephants (Elephas maximas). Vet. Rec., 99 (2): 28-29.

Racaniello, V.R., (2001). Picornaviridae: The viruses and their replication. In: Fields Virology, third ed. Lippincott Williams & Wilkins, pp. 685–722.

Radostits, O.M.; Blood, D.C. and Gay, C.C. (1994). Veterinary Medicine, 8th Edn., Educational Low-Priced scheme. Bailliere Tindall, London, pp. 965-973.

Rai, A. (1980a). Subtyping of foot-and-mouth disease isolate types O and Asia 1 recovered from field outbreaks in India. Indian. J. Anim. Sci., 50, 164-168.

Rai, A. (1980b). A comparative study of the micro-complement fixation and micro neutralization tests in the subtyping of foot and mouth disease virus. Indian. J. Anim. Sci., 50: 961-965.

Rai, A. and Lahiri, D.K. (1981).A micro- enzyme linked labeled immunosorbent assay (Micro-ELISA) for the detection of foot-and-mouth disease virus antigen and antibody. Acta Virol., 25: 49-52.

Ramakant Ahuja, K.L.; Prasad, S.; Tewari, S.C. and Sharma, V.K. (1980). Distribution of foot-and-mouth disease virus in North-West India. Haryana Veterinarian, 19: 144-146.

Rao, B.U. (1989). Development, production and application of vaccines in FMD control in India. In: Progress in Vaccinology, Vol. 2., Talwar, G.P. (Ed.), Springer Verlag , New York Inc., pp. 283-290.

Rasmussen, T.B.; Uttenthal, A.; de Stricker, K.; Belak, S and Storgaard, T. (2003). Development of a novel quantitative real-time RT-PCR assay for the simultaneous detection of all serotypes of foot-and-mouth disease virus. Arch Virol., 148: 2005-2021.

Reid, S.; Ferris, N.; Hutchings G.; Zhang Z.; Belsham, G. and Alexandersen, S. (2002). Detection of all seven serotypes of foot-and-mouth disease virus by real-time, fluorogenic reverse transcription polymerase chain reaction assay. J. Virol. Methods, 105 : 67–80.

Reid, S.M.; Parida, S.; King, D.P.; Hutchings, G.H.; Shaw, A.E.; Ferris, N.P.; Zhang, Z.; Hillerton, J.E. and Paton, D.J. (2006). Utility of automated real-time RT-PCR for the detection of foot-and-mouth disease virus excreted in milk. Vet. Res., 37 (1): 121–132.

Reid, S.M.; Ferris, N.P.; Hutchings, G.H.; Samuel, A.R. and Knowles, N.J. (2000). Primary diagnosis of foot-and-mouth disease by reverse transcription polymerase chain reaction. J. Virol. Methods, 89: 167–176.

Reid, S.M.; Forsyth, M.A.; Hutchings, G.H. and Ferris, N. P. (1998). Comparison of reverse transcription polymerase chain reaction, enzyme linked immunosorbent assay and virus isolation for the routine diagnosis of foot and- mouth disease. J. Virol. Methods, 80: 213–217

Reid, S.M.; Grierson, S.S.; Ferris, N.P.; Hutchings, G.H. and Alexandersen, S. (2003). Evaluation of automated RT-PCR to accelerate the laboratory diagnosis of foot-and-mouth disease virus. J. Virol. Methods, 107 (2): 129–139.

Reid, S.M.; Hutchings, G.H.; Ferris, N.P. and De Clercq, K. (1999). Diagnosis of foot-and-mouth disease by RTPCR: evaluation of primers for serotypic characterisation of viral RNA in clinical samples. J. Virol. Methods, 83: 113–123.

Revenson, S. and Segura, M. (1963). Multiplication of foot-and-mouth disease virus in roller tube culture BHK-21 cells of hamster kidney. Rev. Invest. Canad., 18: 293-299.

Rodriguez, A.; Nunez, J.I.; Nolasco, G.; Ponz, F.; Sobrino, F. and De Blas, C. (1994). Direct PCR detection of foot-and-mouth disease virus. J. Virol. Methods, 47: 345–349.

Roeder, L.P. and Le Blanc Smith, P.M. (1987). Detection and typing of foot-and-mouth disease virus by enzyme linked immunosorbent assay: a sensitive,rapid and reliable technique for primary diagnosis. Res. Vet. Sci., 43: 225-232.

Rossi, M.S.; Sadir, A.M.; Schudel, A.A. and Palma, E.L. (1988). Detection of foot and mouth disease virus with DNA probe in bovine esophageal pharyngeal fluid. Arch. Virol., 99: 67-74.

Rus, Epidemiol. & Infect., 114: 1-13.

Rweyemamu, M. M. (1982). Developments in the biochemical and immunoassays assessment of foot-and-mouth antigen. In: Abstracts, 1st Internationals conference on the impact of viral disease on the development of Latin American countries and Caribbean region. Rio de Janeiro, Brazil, pp 78-79.

Rweyemamu, M. M. (1984). Antigenic variation in foot-and-mouth disease: Studies based on the virus neutralization reaction. J. Biol. Stand., 12: 323-337.

Rweyemamu, M. M.; Booth, J.C.; Head, M. and Pay, T.W.F. (1978).Micro neutralization tests for serological typing and subtyping of FMD virus strains. J. Hyg. Camb., 81: 107-123.

Ryan, M.D.; Belsham, G.J. and King, A.M.Q. (1989). Specificity of enzyme substrate interaction in foot-and-mouth disease virus polyprotein processing. Virology, 173: 35-45.

Ryan, M.D.; King A.M. and Thomas, G.P. (1991). Cleavage of foot-and-mouth disease virus polyprotein is mediated by residues located within a 19 amino acid sequence. J. Gen. Virol., 72: 2727-2732.

Saiki, R.K.; Scharf, S.J.: Faloona, A.F.; Mullis, K.B.; Erlich, H. and Arnheim, N. (1985). Enzymatic amplification of â- goblin genomic sequence and restriction site analysis for the diagnosis of sickle cell anemia. Science, 230: 1350-1354.

Salt, J.S. (1993). The carrier state in foot and mouth disease: an immunological review. Br. Vet. J., 149: 207-/223.

Sammin, D.J.; Paton, D.J.; Parida, S.; Ferris, N.P.; Hutchings, G.H.; Reid, S.M.; Shaw, A.E.; Holmes, C.; Gibson, D.; Corteyn, M.; Knowles, N.J.; Valarcher, J.-F.; Hamblin, P.A.; Fleming, L.; Gwaze, G. and Sumption, K.J. (2007). Evaluation of laboratory tests for SAT serotypes of foot-and-mouth disease virus with specimens collected from convalescent cattle in Zimbabwe. Vet. Rec., 160 (19): 647–654.

Sarma, D.K.; Dutta, P.K. and Harzarika, A.K. (1992). Foot-and-mouth disease in North Eastern India during 1991. Virus Information Exchange Newsletter for South East Asia and the Western Pacific., 9: 63-64.

Schweiger, B.; Zadow, I.; Heckler, R.; Timm, H. and Pauli, G. (2000). Application of a fluorogenic PCR assay for typing and subtyping of influenza viruses in respiratory samples. J. Clin. Microbiol., 38 (4): 1552–1558.

Sellers, R.F. (1955). Growth and titration of the viruses of foot-and-mouth disease and vesicular stomatitis in kidney monolayer tissue cultures. Nature, 176: 121-124.

Sellers, R.F. (1971). Quantitative aspects of the spread of foot and mouth disease. Vet. Bull., 41: 431-439.

Shaw, A.E.; Reid, S.M.; King, D.P.; Hutchings. G.H. and Ferris, N.P. (2004). Enhanced laboratory diagnosis of foot and mouth disease by real-time polymerase chain reaction. Rev. sci. tech. Off. int. Epiz., 23 (3): 1003-1009

Snowden, W.A. (1966). Growth of foot-and-mouth disease virus in monolayer cultures of calf thyroid cells. Nature, 210: 1079-1080.

Sobrino, F and E. Domingo. (2001) . Foot-and-mouth disease in Europe. EMBO Rep., 2: 459–461.

Stanley Tam.; Alfonso Clavijo.; Eric, K. Engelhard. and Mark, C. T. (2009). Fluorescence based multiplex real-time PCR arrays for the detection and serotype determination of foot-and-mouth disease virus. J. Virol. Methods, 161: 183-191.

Strohmaier, K.; Franze, R. and Adam, K. H. (1982) Location and characterization of the antigenic portion of the foot-and-mouth disease virus immunizing protein, J. Gen. Virol., 59: 295-306.

Sutmoller, P. (1992) Vesicular Diseases, Foreign Animal Diseases, Committee on Foreign Animal Diseases of the United States Animal Health Association, VA, Richmond. pp. 368–382.

Tamilselvan, R.P.; De Sanyal, A. and Pattnaik, B. (2009): Genetic transitions of Indian serotype O Foot and Mouth Disease Virus isolates responsible for field outbreaks during 2001-2009: A brief note: OIE/ FAO Reference laboratories network meeting: 23rd to 27th November, 2009. New Delhi. pp 11- 13.

Tewari, S.C.; Singh, I.P.; Ramakant; Sharma, V.K.; Pandey, R. and Prasad, S. (1975). A note on the incidence and distribution of foot-and-mouth disease virus types in north-west India. Indian J. Anim. Sci., 45: 159-60.

Traub, E. and Mohalman, H. (1943). Foot-and- mouth disease typing with complement fixation test first communication. Experiment with serum and antigen of guinea pigs. Zentr Bacteriol Parasitenk Orig Abt I., 150: 289-300 (cited by Bachrach, 1968)

Vallee, H. and Carre, H. (1922). Sur la pluralite' du virus aphteux. Comp. Rend. Acad. Sci., 174: 1498 (cited in by Fred Brown, 2003)

Vangrysperre, W. and De Clercq, K. (1996). Rapid and sensitive polymerase chain reaction based detection and typing of foot-and-mouth disease virus in clinical samples and cell culture isolates, combined with other genomically and/or symptomically related viruses. Arch. Virol., 141: 331-344.

Verma, N.D. and Sarma, D.K. (1997). Note on foot-and-mouth disease in Mithun in Arunachal Pradesh. Indian. J. Virol., 13(1): 75-76

Vosloo, W.; Boshoff, K.; Darka, R. and Bastos, A. (2002). The possible role that buffalo played in the recent outbreaks of foot-and-mouth disease in South Africa. Ann. N.Y. Acad. Sci., 969: 187-190.

Waldmann, O. and Pape, J. (1920). Die Kuenstilche Uebertragung der Maulund Klauenseuche auf das Meerschweinchen. Berl. Tierarztl.Wschr., 36: 519-520. (Cited by Brown, F.2003, Virus Res., 91:3-7.

Waldmann, O. and Trautwein, K. (1926). Experimentelle Untersuchungen ueber die Pluralitet des Maul-und Klauenseuche Virus. Berl. Iterarztl. Wschr., 42: 569-571. (Cited by Brown, F.2003, Virus Res., 91: 3-7.

Woodbury, R. L. (1995). A review of the possible mechanisms for the persistence of foot-and-mouthdisease vi Dutta, P.K.; Sharma, G. and Das, S.K. (1984). Occurrence of foot-and-mouth disease and distribution of virus type in the hill states of North Eastern region of India. Indian J. Anim. Sci., 4: 117-118.

Zhang, Z. and Alexandersen, S. (2003). Detection of carrier cattle and sheep persistently infected with foot-and-mouth disease virus by a rapid real-time RT-PCR assay. J. Virol. Methods, 111: 95-100.

□□□

Chapter 8

Bovine Tuberculosis : An Overview

YOSEF DENEKE
Assistant Professor, Jimma University
School of Veterinary Medicine, Ethopia

Bovine tuberculosis is an infectious disease caused by *Mycobacterium bovis* (M. bovis) characterized by formation of tubercle in tissue/ organ of the animal. It remains as one of the most devastating diseases of cattle in developing countries throughout the world (Berrada and Banajas- Rojas, 1995). The disease is important not only because of its determinant effect on animal production but also for public health reasons (Radostits *et al*, 1994). Infection in humans occurs largely through children consuming infected milk but it can also be spread through inhalation . Most species of domestic and wild animals are susceptible to *Mycobacterium bovis*. Cattle, goats and pigs are more susceptible while sheep and horse have high natural resistance (Radostits *et al.*, 2000). Infected cattle are the main source of infection for other cattle. The bacteria are excreted in the exhaled air, in sputum, milk, urine, vaginal and uterine discharge (Radostits *et al.*, 2000). Diagnosis of bovine tuberculosis in developing countries is mainly done by tuberculin test and post mortem examination as bacteriology involve higher cost (Regassa and Ameni, 2000).

Etiology

Bovine tuberculosis (BTB) is an infectious disease of cattle mainly caused by *Mycobacterium bovis (M.bovis)* and characterized by progressive development of tubercles in any tissue /organ of the body (Clark, 1998). *M. bovis* is genetically very similar to *Mycobacterium tuberculosis* (*M. tuberculosis*), the major pathogen that causes human tuberculosis. It is one of the species of mycobacteria belonging to the *Mycobacterium tuberculosis* complex comprising *M. tuberculosis, M. bovis, M. microti, M. Canetti* and *M .africanum* (Collin and Grange, 1983; Pritchard, 1988). Tuberculous mycobacteria are alcohol-acid resistant, non spore forming, gram positive bacilli. These mycobacterial organisms are resistant to many disinfectants, desiccation and other adverse environmental factors as their cell wall have high lipid contents (Ernstand Hirsh, 1999).

Epidemiology

Bovine tuberculosis occurs in every country of the world and is major important disease in dairy cattle. It can be occurred in all species including man. It is important not only for public health reasons but also its detrimental effects on animal production (Radostits *et al.*, 1989).The main source of infection of tubercle bacilli is tuberculous individuals. Humans perpetuate M. tuberculosis. Where as cattle and chickens perpetuates *M. bovis* and *M. avium,* respectively (Ernst and Hirsh, 1999). Radostits *et al.* (1989) on its turn indicated that the infected animals are the main source of infection. The organisms are excreted in the exhaled air, in sputum, feces, milk, urine, vaginal and uterine discharges.

Common entry of the organisms is effected by inhalation or ingestion. Inhalation is almost the invariably portal of entry in housed cattle and even in those that are at pasture. It is considered to be the principal mode of transmission. Infection by ingestion is obviously more likely at pasture when feces contaminate the feed and communal drinking water. Drinking of infected milk by young animals is also one of the commonest methods by which tuberculosis is spread (Radostits *et al.*, 2000).

Tuberculosis had at times presented one of the deadly threats to human being. Between 1700 and 1900, almost every one form the temperate region was infected with tuberculosis; in certain regions every fourth death was due to tuberculosis (Kleebeg, 1984). Because of the corrective measures applied the disease has practically disappeared from most of the developed countries, remaining an increasingly serious problem of the developing world.

In developed countries bovine tuberculosis has eradicated or in advanced stage of control, while in several developing countries the situation has not improved or prevalence is increasing. Almost all western European countries reported a prevalence of bovine tuberculosis infection lower than 0.1%. In the western hemisphere, Canada and the US have reduced the infection rate to very low levels. In the US in1969, 0.06% of 4.5 million cattle examined react to tuberculosis. In Latin America, Costarica, Cuba, Jamaica, Panama, Uruguay and Venezuela have national bovine tuberculosis programs (Pedro andSzyfres, 2001).

Public Health Importance

Bovine tuberculosis is not only the infection of animals but also it affects human beings in both developed and developing countries (Pedron and Szyfres, 2001). In England, where the bovine tuberculosis eradication and milk pasteurization was followed, 63 patients of 5,021 (1.12%) were tuberculosis positive of animal origin from the year 1977 to 1979. Of these cases, 27 (42.85%) had pulmonary tuberculosis and 36 (57.14%) had extra pulmonary tuberculosis. In Slovakia, 52 human cases caused by the bovine bacilli were recorded during the period 1979-1983, 10 to 15 years after the eradication of bovine tuberculosis (Burjanova and Nagyova, 1985). Where as inGermany during the period 1960 s when the bovine tuberculosis in cattle was high, 45 % of the tuberculous adenitis cases in children were caused by *M. bovis*. In the US at the beginning of 20th century, up to 20% of human tuberculosis was attributed to M. bovis; in 1980, barely 0.1% of human tuberculosis was so attributed (Good and Snider, 1980). In countries where milk is routinely boiled, as in Latin America, the incidence of infection by *M. bovis* has been always low. Nevertheless, the pulmonary and the extra pulmonary forms of human tuberculosis of animal origin have continued to be a problem in areas where the prevalence of infection in cattle is high. This is because not all milk consumed is boiled; many products are prepared from un pastured milk; and cases of infection are contracted via aerosols. In Peru, a study of 853 strains of pulmonary tuberculosis identified 38 (4.45%) as *M.bovis* (Fernandez, Salazar *et al.*, 1983). Sinha (1994) estimated that *M. bovis* accounts for 30% of tuberculosis in children and up to 10% of the extra pulmonary form of tuberculosis in human being as a whole in the border area between Mexico and USA.

Clinical Sign and Pathogenesis

Clinical signs

Although signs referable to localization in a particular organ usually attract attention to the possible occurrence of tuberculosis, some general signs are also evident. Some cows with extensive milliary tubercular lesions are clinically normal. But progressive emaciation unassociated with other sign should always arouse suspension of tuberculosis. A capricious appetite and fluctuating temperature are also commonly associated with the disease; affected animals become docile and sluggish (Radostits, *et al.*, 1989). Pulmonary involvement is characterized by chronic coughing due to bronco pneumonia. The cough is never loud or paroxysmal, occurring only once or twice at a time and is low, suppressed and moist. In the advanced stages when much lung has been destroyed, dyspnea with increased rate and depth of respiration becomes apparent. Involvement of the bronchial lymph nodes may cause dyspnea because of the constriction of the air passages, and enlargement of the mediastinal lymph node is commonly associated with recurrent and then persistent ruminal tympani (Radostits, *et al.*, 1989). The most common sign of alimentary involvement are caused by pressure of enlarged lymph node on surrounding organs. Rarely tuberculous ulcers of the small intestine cause diarrhea. Retropharyngeal lymph node enlargement causes dyspnea and noisy breathing due to pharyngeal obstruction (Ernst and Hirsh, 1999).

Pathogenesis

Infection of tuberculosis begins with development of tubercle bacilli in the lung, pharyngeal or intestinal mucus membranes. In previously exposed animals, local multiplication occurs as macrophage on the scene ingests the organisms. Resistance to phagositc killing (mycosides, phospholipids and sulfolipids apparently protect tubercle bacilli against phagocytic killing) continued intracellular and extra cellular multiplication. An inflammatory response (wax D an auto lysate of *M .tuberculosis* activates macrophages and induce granulomatous lesions) involving largely histocytes and monocytes develop around the focus of the proliferating organisms. Infected host cells and bacteria reach draining lymph nodes where proliferation and inflammatory response continued (Ernst and Hirsh, 1999). After the first week, cell mediated immune reaction begin to modify the host response from essentially a foreign body reaction to a reaction characteristics of infectious granulomas. Infected macrophage secret IL-12 a cytokine responsible for stimulating $CD4^t$ T_{H1} lymphocytes to produce gamma interferon (INF), granulocyte monocytecolony stimulating factors (GM-CSF), and migration inhibition factor (MIF), which attract and activate macrophages. Activated macrophages acquired the capacity to kill mycobacteria (Ernst and Hirsh, 1999). Their efficiency in doing so depends on the adequacy of the immune response and the virulence of the bacteria. Stimulated $CD4T_{H1}$ as well as gamma-delta T lymphocytes lyse mycobacteria containing macrophages. Recognition of infected macrophages is probably due to increased expression of "stress" proteins by the infected macrophage. Epitheloid cells appeared among the macrophages. They often become the predominant cells. A third rarer cells in the lesion are the giant cells which are probably macrophage derivatives. At the center the lesion, caseation necrosis develops. A function of the allergic state it may proceed calcification or liquefactions (Managhan *et al.*, 1994).

Diagnosis

Bovine tuberculosis caused by *M. bovis* can be diagnosed both in life animals and after death. It can be diagnosed by clinical signs and primarily on the basis delayed hypersensitivity reaction; after death by post mortem, histopathological and bacteriological examinations (OIE, 1996).The symptoms of bovine TB depend on the organs involved and the extent of the lesion. It is usually a progressive disease accompanied by marked weight loss, decreased milk production and weakness. Duration of the clinical course is measured by weeks and months. Gradual emaciation, enlargement of lymph nodes, coughing intermittently and increment of body temperature are some of the manifested clinical signs (Leper *et al.*, 1977). Because of the chronic nature of the disease and multiplicity of signs caused by variable location of the infection, TB is difficult to diagnose on clinical examination (Radostits *et al.*, 2000). Tuberculin tests have been used for diagnosis of tuberculosis in cattle. It is the standard diagnostic test for bovine tuberculosis (Merchant, 1983). Tuberculin is the name given to extract of *M. bovis, M. tuberculosis* and *M. avium* which is used to identify those animals which are previously exposed to mycobacterium organisms. Several types of tuberculin have been used for this purpose but the most important one is the purified protein derivatives (PPD). Its major antigenic component is probably heat shocked protein (Tizard, 1996).

When PPD is injected intra dermally in to a normal animal, there is no significant local response. But when it is inoculated in to exposed animals, there is an allergic skin reaction which is typically the delayed type of hyper sensitivity reaction (Klein, 1990; Ragassa, 1999; Radostits, 2000). Comparative intra dermal tuberculin test is one of the most important method of tuberculin tests which is used to differentiate between animals infected with the mammalian tuberculosis (*M. bovis* and *M. tuberculosis*) and those sensitized to tuberculin due to exposure to other mycobacteia or related genera (Mananghan *et al.*, 1994). Tentative diagnosis of bovine tuberculosis can be made on the detection of gross lesions at necropsy. Careful examination of lymph nodes, lung, intestine, liver and spleen can result 95% of the cattle with macroscopic lesion (Comer, 1994). On gross necropsy examination, tuberculosis may be provisionally diagnosed when gaseous or calcified foci are observed in various tissues of the body; but this is difficult in the initial stage of the disease or when the changes are non specific (OIE, 1996). Blood based laboratory tests have become available corresponding to immunity are the lymphocyte proliferative assay (LPA) and the gamma interferon assay (GIA) while the enzyme linked immune sorbant assay (ELISA) corresponds to humeral immunity. Serological tests are less important for the diagnosis of BTB because antibody response to *M. bovis* is poor until there is advanced disease (OIE, 1996).

Control and Prevention

Prevention of animals from infection can be done by testing the introducing animal by tuberculin test assuming the present herd is free of bovine tuberculosis. Prevention of human from infection by *M. bovis* consists of the pasteurization of milk, vaccination with BCG and above all, control and eradication of bovine tuberculosis (Pedron and Szyfres, 2001). The only rational approach to reduce and eradicate losses produced by the infection in cattle preventing human cases caused by *M. bovis* is establishing a control and eradication program for bovine tuberculosis. Control in a herd rests on removal of the infected animals, prevention of spread of infection and avoidance of further introduction of the disease (Radostits *et al.*, 1989). Application of tuberculin test and slaughter of reactor animals has given excellent results in all counties that have undertaken eradication campaigns. At present many developed countries are free or practically free of B. tuberculosis (Pedron and Szyfres, 2001). In developing countries, the inability of governments to compensate owners for the destruction of reactor hinders establishment of eradication programs and makes it necessary to find other incentives, such as surcharge on milk. Campaigns should be begun in regions of lower prevalence, where replacing reactor animal is easier and using the comparative intra dermal tuberculin test would be better in areas where *Mycobacterium para tuberculosis* and *Mycobacterium avium* are more prevalent diseases (Radostits *et al.*, 1989). Controlling tuberculosis caused by *M. bovis* in its principal reservoir, cattle, is the best method of preventing transmission to other species, including man.

Vaccination may consider under certain circumstance particularly when an eradication program can not be instituted for some time but it is desired to decrease the incidence the disease. BCG vaccine is the only method available for field level, the vole acid-fast vaccine varying too much in virulence. How ever it has several disadvantages; Vaccination is carried out by subcutaneous injection of 50-100 ml vaccine and large and un slightly lumps appear at the injection site; injection by the other alternative intra venous route is attended by risk of sever systemic reactions. As the immunity is not strong, vaccinated animals should not be submitted to sever exposure (Radostits *et al.*, 1989).

Treatment with anti-tuberculosis drugs, particularly, isoniazid takes many months, on the top of its costyness, can produce drug resistance to *M. bovis* strains, and the result is un certain (Pedron and Szyfres, 2001).

References

Acha, P.N. and Szyfres, B. (1987): Zoonotic tuberculosis. In Zoonoses and communicable diseases common to man and animals, 2nd ed. Pan American. Health Organization (PAHO), World Health Organization (WHO), Washington, D.C

Adugna, W. (2005): Bovine TB: Epidemiological survey in specialized and small holder dairy farms in and around Dredawa, Eastern Ethiopia . DVM thesis, FVM, Addis AbabaUniversity , Debrezeit , Ethiopia . pp.490.

Aklilu,E. (2005): Bovine TB: Prevalence in small holder dairy farms and its public health implications in Adama, central Ethiopia . DVM thesis, FVM, Addis AbabaUniversity , Debrezeit , Ethiopia . pp.467-468.

Alemayehu, M. (2003): Country Pasture/Forage Resource Profiles. Suttie J.M., Reynolds S.G. (eds.). 1–36. http://www.fao.org

Alemu T. (1992): Bovine tuberculosis in Ethiopia. Tropical animal health and production. University of Edinburgh, Centre for Tropical Veterinary Medicine, UK.

Ameni, G. (1996): Bovine TB: Evaluation of diagnostic tests, prevalence and zoonotic importance. DVM Thesis, FVM, Addis AbabaUniversity , Debrezeit , Ethiopia . pp. 226.

Ameni, G., Roger F. (1998): Study on the epidemiology of bovine tuberculosis in dairy farms (Debre-Zeit and Ziway, Ethiopia). In: Proceeding of the 12th Conference of the Ethiopian Veterinary Association (EVA), Addis Ababa, Ethiopia. pp 13–19.

Ameni, G., Amenu, K. and Tibbo, M. (2002): Bovine tuberculosis prevalence and risk factor assessment in cattle and cattle owners in Wuchale-jida District,central Ethiopia. Int. J.appl. Vet. Med. **1**, pp. 17-26

Ameni, G., Amenu, K., Tibbo M. (2003a): Bovine tuberculosis: prevalence and risk factors assessment in cattle and cattle owners in Wuchale-Jida district, Central Ethiopia. International Journal of Applied Research in Veterinary Medicine, **1**, pp. 17–25.

Ameni, G., Bonner P., Tibbo M. (2003b): Across-sectional study of bovine tuberculosis in selected dairy farms in Ethiopia. International Journal of Applied Research in Veterinary Medicine, **1**, Pp. 85–97.

Ameni, G., Aseffa, A., Engers, H., Young, D. B., Hewinson, G. R., Vordermeier, M.H. (2006): Cattle husbandry is a predominant factor affecting the pathology of bovine

Ameni, G., Aseffa, A., Engers, H., Young, D. B., Hewinson, G. R., Vordermeier, M.H. (2007): High prevalence and Increased Sevirity of Pathology of Bovine tuberculosis in Holstein Compared to Zebu Breeds under Field Cattle Husbandry in Central Ethiopia. Clinical and Vaccine immunology, American society for Microbiology. Pp. 1356-1361.

Amenu, K(2002): Bovine TB: Prevalence and public health implications in small Holder farms in Wuchale Jida district central Ethiopia. DVM thesis, FVM, Addis AbabaUniversity, Debrezeit, Ethiopia. Pp.355-356.

Assegd, B., Lubke-Becker, A., Lemma, E., Tadeld, K. and Britton, S. (2000): Bovine tuberculosis: a cross-sectional and epidemiological study in and around Addis Ababa. Bull. Anim.Hlth prod. Afr., **48**, Pp.71-80.

Asseged B., Lubke-Beker A., Lemma E., Kiros T., Britton S. (2001): Bovine tuberculosis: A cross sectional and epidemiological study in and around Addis Ababa.

Ayele W.Y., Neill S.D., Zinsstag J., Weiss M.G., Pavlik I. (2004): Bovine tuberculosis: an old disease but a new threat to Africa. International Journal of Tuberculosis and Lung Disease, **8**, 924–937.

Barwinnek, F., Taylor, N.M. (1996): Assessment of the socio-economic importance of BTB in Turkey and WHO (1993): Report of WHO working group on zoonotic TB (*M. bovis*) with the participation of FAO. Geneva, Pp. 1-26

Belay, M. (2000): Cross-sectional study on bovine TB in small holders dairy farms and its implication in Fitche town, Northern Shoa .DVM thesis, FVM, Addis AbabaUniversity, Debrezeit, Ethiopia. Pp. 308.

Berroda, J. & Barajas–Rojas J.A. (1995): Control of bovine TB In developing countries. In: Mycobacterium bovis infection in animals & humans (C.O. Theen & J.H. Steele, eds). Iowa state University press, Amess , Iowa , Pp. 159-166

Bulletin of Animal Health and Production in Africa, **48**, 71–80.

Clarke, C.F. (1998). Tuberculosis. In Aiello, S.E. (Ed) the merk veterinary manual 8th*ed.* Merk and Co.,NC.USA.

Collins, C.H. and Grnage, S.M. (1983): A review; The bovine tuberculosis. Journal on Applied Bacteriology. **55**, pp.13-39.

Collins, C.H. and Grange, J.M. (1985): Organization and practice in tuberculosis bacteriology, Butter Worth London pp. 281.

Comer, L.A. (1994): Post mortem Diagnosis of *Mycobacterium bovis* infection in cattle. Vet. Microbiol. **40**, 53-65.

Cook, A.J.C.,Tuchili, L.M., Buve, A., Foster, S.D., Godfrey- Fausett, P., Pandy, G.S., and McAdam, K.P.W.J. (1996): Human and bovine tuberculosisin the Monze District of Zambia- a cross-sectional study. Br. Vet.J., **152**, pp. 37-46.

Daborn, C.J., Grange J.M., Kazwala R.R. (1996): Bovine tuberculosis cycle: an African prospective. Journal of Applied Bacteriology, **81**, pp. 275–325.

Dejene, A.T. (1998): Bovine TB: Evaluation of diagnostic tests Prevalence and Zoonotic Importance: DVM Thesis, FVM, Addis AbabaUniversity , Debrezeit , Ethiopia . pp. 256.

Ernst, L.B. and Hirsh, D.C. (1999): Mycobacterium species, The agent of Animal tuberculosis. In: Veterinary microbiology, Blackwell science, Ltd, Blackwell publishing Campany. pp 158-164.

FAO (1967): Report to the Government of Ethiopia. Food and Agriculture Organization, Veterinary Service and Disease Control. Animal health service Rome, Italy.

FAO (1972): Report to the Government of Ethiopia. Food and Agriculture Organization veterinary service and disease control. Animal health service, Rome, Italy.

Good, R.C.and Snider, J.R.,(1980): Isolation of nontuberculous Mycobacteria in the United States, J.infect Dis pp 829-833.

Hailemariam, S. (1975): A brief analysis of activities of meat inspection and quarantine division. Department of Veterinary Service, MoA, Addis Ababa, Ethiopia.

Kazwala, R.R., Kusiluka, L.J.M., Jiva, S.F.H (1998): Isolation of Mycobacterium species from raw milk of pastorial cattle in the Southerland High Lands of Tanzania. Trop. Anim. Hlth prod., **30** pp 233- 239

Kebede, E. (2005): Bovine TB: Addis Ababa Dairy farms. DVM thesis, FVM, Addis AbabaUniversity , Debrezeit , Ethiopia . pp466.

Kiros, T. (1998): Epidemiology and zoonotic importance of bovine tuberculosis in selected sites of Eastern Shewa Ethiopia. MSc. Thesis, Faculty of Veterinary Medicine, Addis Ababa, University and Freie Universitat, Berlin, Germany.

Kleeberg, H.H. (1984): Human TB of bovine origin in relation to public health. Scientific and Technical Review, Organization for International Epizootic. **3**, pp.226.

Klein, J. (1990): Immunology, 1st ed., Black Well Scientific Publication, Boston. pp 451-459.

Laval, G. and Ameni, G. (2004): Prevalence of bovine tuberculosis in zebu cattle under traditional animal husbandry in Boji District of western Ethiopia. Rev. Med. Vet. **155:** Pp. 152-159

Lepper, A.W.D., Pearson, C.W. and Corner, L.A. (1977): Anergy to tuberculin in beef cattle. Aus. Vet.J.**53**, 214-216.

Liss,G.M, Wong, h., Kittle.D.C., Simor, A Naus,M., Martiquet,p.and Misener C.R. (1997): Occuptional exposure to Mycobacterium bovis infection in deer and elk in Ontario . Can J.public health. **85**, pp.326-329

MoA (1984): Livestock Sector Review. Annex.1. Ministry of Agriculture, Addis Ababa, Ethiopia.

Managhan, M.L., Collins, J.D., Kazada, J.F. and Quinn, P.J.(1994): The tuberculin test.Veterinary Microbioly,**40**, pp 111-124.

Merchant, I.A. (1983): Veterinary Bacteriology and Virology, 7th ed.,CBS Publisher. pp 441-466.

OIE (1996): Manual Techniques and requirement for biological products. **1**, pp .287-294

Pedron, N.A. and Szyfres, B. (2001): Zoonosis and Communicable Diseases to common man and Animals. 3th ed., Pan American Health Organization, Washington, U.S.A. pp 283-296.

Pritchard, D.G. (1988): Century of bovine TB from 1888-1988 consequence and controversy. Journal of comparative pathology vol **99**:Pp.357-399.

Putt, S.N.H., Shaw, A.P.M., Woods, A.J., Tylor, L. and James, A.D. (1988). Veterinary epidemiology and economics in Africa: A manual for use in the design and appraisal of livestock health policy, 2nd ed. International livestock center for Africa (ILCA) Manual No.5.ILCA

Radostits, O.M., Gay, C.C., Blood D.C., Hinchelift K.W. (2000): Disease caused by bacteria – *Mycobacterium*. In: Veterinary Medicine: A Text Book of Disease of Cattle, Sheep, Pig, Goat and Horses. 9th ed. Harcourt Publisher Ltd., London. pp. 909–918.

Radostits, O.M., Blood, D.C. and Gay, C.C., (1994): Disease caused by mycobacterium species. In Veterinary medicine: a textbook of the disease of cattle, sheep, pigs, goats and horses, 8th Ed. Bailliere Tidall, London, 830-850.

Redi, N. (2003): Prevalence of bovine TB and its Zoonotic implications in Asela town, Southern Ethiopia. DVM thesis, FVM, Addis AbabaUniversity, Debrezeit, Ethiopia. pp. 397.

Regassa, A. (1999): Preliminary study on bovie TB. In Wolyta Sodo , Southern, Ethiopia . DVM Thesis, FVM, Addis AbabaUniversity, Debrezeit , Ethiopia . pp. 268-269

Regassa, A. and Ameni, G. (2000): Sensitivity and Specificity of single intra dermal tuberculin test at the cervical and caudal folds in Zebu cattle in Ethiopia; In Indian Journal of Animal Science, **71**. pp.325-327.

Regassa A. (2005): Study on *Mycobacterium bovis* in animals and human in and around Fiche, North Shewa zone, Ethiopia. MSc. Theses. Faculty of Veterinary Medicine, Addis AbabaUniversity, Debre-Zeit, Ethiopia

Seifert, H.S.H. (1996): Contact diseases caused by actonomyseta. In tropical animal health, 2nd ed. Kluwer Academic, Dordrecht, the Netherlands, 343-349.

Shitaye, J.E., Getahun B., Alemayehu T., Skoric M., Treml F., Fictum P., Vrbas V., Pavlikl. (2006): A prevalence study of bovine tuberculosis by using abattoir meat

Tizard, D.E.R.(1996): Veterinary Immunology. An introduction, 5th ed., Harcourt Brace and Company Asia PTE Ltd., India. pp 55-65.

UN, HIV/AIDS (2001): Population impacts and policies population Division Department of economics and social Affairs United Nations.

World Organization for Animal Health (OIE) (2000): Bovine TB.In Manual of standards for diagnostic test and vaccines, 4th ed. OIE. Paris. pp. 451-463.

Wudie, A. (2003): Preliminary study on bovine TB in Northern Municipality Abattoir, Central Ethiopia. DVM thesis, FVM, Addis AbabaUniversity, Debrezeit, Ethiopia. Pp.370.

Yehualashet, T. (1995): Status of bovine tuberculosis in Ethiopia. In Mycobacterium bovis infection in animals and humans (C.O. Thoen and J.H. Steel, eds) Iowa State University Press, Ames, Iowa.pp 273-278.

Zinsstag J., Kazwala R.R., CadmusI., Ayanwale L. (2006a): *Mycobacterium bovis* in Africa. In: Thoen C.O., Steele J.H. Gilsdorf M.F. (eds.): *Mycobacterium bovis* Infection in Animals and Humans. 2nd ed. Blackwell Publishing Professional, Ames, Iowa, USA. pp199–210.

□□□

Chapter 9

Antigen Based Diagnosis of Paratuberculosis

RAJIB DEB[1] AND VIJAY KUMAR SAXENA[2]
[1] Scientist, Project Directorate on Cattle, Indian Council of Agricultural Research Meerut Cantt-250 001, Uttar Pradesh, India
[2] Scientist, CSWRI, Avikanagar (Rajasthan)

Paratuberculosis is a chronic infectious disease of domestic animals as well as some wild ruminants and laboratory animals are also susceptible for the same. The identification of the etiological agent is attributed to F.W. Twort, who in 1912 shown that the causative agent of the disease can be cultivated in vitro and in 1914 experimentally it was proved that *Mycobacterium avium subsp. paratuberculosis* (MAP) is the main causative agent of the disease. The organism is acid as well as alcholfast, slow growing, fastidious bacterium requiring exogenous mycobactin for its in vitro growth (Chiodini *et al.,* 1984). This organism has also been reported to be associated with cases of Crohn's disease, a chronic fatal multifactorial inflammatory bowel disease in humans (Ghadiali *et al.,* 2004; Naser *et al.,* 2004). Paratuberculosis is an enzootic disease on the B list of the Office des International Epizootes ('OIE').Disease causes huge production losses and has high impact on animal industry, where premature culling, reduces carcass value, reduce weight gain, increase susceptibility to other infection, reduce fertility and milk production as well as feed efficiency. The causative agent, originally named *Mycobacterium enteritidis chronicae pseudo-tuberculosae bovis johne*, was then referred as *Mycobacterium* *paratuberculosis.*The classification of *M.paratuberculosis* has followed classical bacterial lines based on the main criteria of extremely slow growth and the requirement of exogenous mycobactin J. However, some strains of *M.avium* designated wood pigeon mycobacteria require exogenous mycobactin only on primary isolation but later become independent of it on subsequent passage. According to kunze *et al.,* (1992) *Mycobacteria* can be differentiated on the basis of the specific insertion sequence on their genomic DNA. *M.paratuberculosis* possesses the specific insertion sequence IS 900 and the *M.avium* can be divided into two distinct biotypes according to the presence of IS 901. Thorel *et al.,* (1990) proposed a classification of *M.avium* based on a large number of biochemical tests into three subspecies, viz., *M.avium* subspecies *paratuberculosis, M.avium* subspecies *avium* and *M.avium* subspecies *silvaticum* (wood pigeon mycobacteria). *M.paratuberculosis,* causative agent of paratuberculosis in the ruminants is now known as *M.avium* ssp. *paratuberculosis* (*M.a.paratuberculosis*) or simply Map, belonging to the *M.avium* complex (MAC) group of organisms. The disease is ubiquitous and distributed throughout the world including India. Numerous reports of the infection are available on cattle, sheep and goats. Motiwala *et al.,* 2004 have reported occurrence of the disease in wild ruminants and birds. Johne's disease causes severe economic losses to the cattle and dairy industry. A survey estimated that 20% of dairy herds in the USA are infected with *M.a.paratuberculosis* resulting in $220 million annual losses. (Wells and Wanger, 2000).

To date no effective therapeutic or vaccine agents are available and early detection along with good management practices are the only ways to control paratuberculosis (Harris and Barletta, 2001). Unfortunately, control programmes are hampered by the lack of simple and efficient diagnostic tests, especially for subclinically infected animals. Serological and cell mediated immunity based assays remain most promising but so far specific immuno-dominant antigens are lacking (Bannantine *et al.,* 2004). A postgenomic analysis of *Mycobacterium avium subsp. Paratuberculosis* proteins identified specific antigens that could potentially improve the diagnosis of paratuberculosis. Currently used antigens for diagnostic tests of *M. avium paratuberculosis* have variable success as regard to specificity and sensitivity. So there is no matter to surprise that presently used conventional methods for diagnosis are inadequate and unreliable. Advance DNA technology has opened a new era for exploring various recombinant antigens of *Mycobacterium avium subsp. Paratuberculosis* which can develop specific and sensitive diagnostic tests.

Conventional Methods for Detection Paratuberculosis Infection

Direct microscopic methods

In direct method, clinical samples are examined for detection of organisms fecal sources are the main route transmission of the disease.staining of fecal samples for detection of acid fast bacilli may reveal mycobacterial bacilli, but the sensitivity of this reaction is very low. It is difficult to distinguish accurately Map from nonpathogenic mycobacteria (saprophytes) in such samples can be difficult , so it having very low specificity.

Culturing of the organism

Collected fecal samples should be treat to kill other organisms than Map , the main constrains with conventional culturing system is that, it takes around 12-16 weeks to detect the growth of colony diverse strain of the species required different growth media for their propagation in in-vitro culture. Clinical samples including feces, tissue samples like-intestine, MLN, SMLN, liver, testes,uder,uterus etc, blood, milk can be used to identify Map from infected animals. Herrold's egg media or modified Lowenstein-jnsen media supplemented with iron chelator especially mycobactin are preffered by diagnostics laboratory to isolate Map (whipple *et al.,* 1991).Map are slow growing organisms takes 8-9 weeks to colonized, they require mycobactin J for their growth, they are acid aswell as alcholfast organism and IS900 Sequence specific PCR. By cultureing techniques we can detect infected animals shedding more than 100 CFU/g of feces . Some disadvantages in this methods are long incubation period (2-4 months), lack of reproductibility organisms can not distribute homogenously in feces.

Radioisotopic culture

In this methods the culture can be radiolabelled with radioisotope indicator system along with antibiotics, permits detection of as few as 3 organism per gram of sample, by this technique we can detect the organisms within few week to few days depending on the load of organisms in the samples some examples of this radiometric culture are -BACTEC 12B and BACTEC460. Main disadvantages with BACTEC method is that- it is more expensive, requirement of sophisticated instrumentation and hazardous complicacy of radioisotope cultures.

Molecular Methods for Diagnosis

PCR based diagnosis

Most progress made in improving diagnosis has been made in direct detection of Map by virtue of the specific sequence ISO 900 (genetic probes) and advent of gene amplification techniques like PCR. Various mycobacteria infection can be diagnosed by PCR (Hawkey, 1994). PCR provides a rapid and specific detection of Map within 24 hours or some cases 2-3 days . It is reported that due to presence of PCR enzyme inhibitor sometime to detect ISO geneprobe become difficults (Stevenson *et al.*, 1997). Again the geneticprobe based on 16s RNA is identical for both *M. paratuberuclosis* and *M. avium* and so it could not be considered as specific probes for paratuberculosis detection. An improved version of immunomagnetic PCR is available for diagnosis of *M.A. paratuberculosis* in milk samples (Grant, 1999).

However PCR is less sensitive than culture when applied to screen clinical samples due to presence of inhibitory substances or non recovery of DNA. Another aspect is nonspecificity of IS900 due to presence of IS900 like sequence in non- Map mycobacteria (Collins, 1996).

Other Molecular Tools

With the development of standarised procedure of PFGE (Pulsed Field Gel Electrophoresis) it is possible to characterised and phylogenetically analysis of Map (Hughes *et al.*, 2001). PFGE revealed two different types of organisms viz., type 1 (pigmented) mainly in sheep and type 2 (nonpigmented) which has broad ranges hosts (Stevenson *et al.,* 2002). Again it is demonstrated that different strain of Map like C1-C5 (cattle), S(sheep) and I(intermediates) have been described by means of RFLP (Restriction Fragment Length Polymorphism) with various enzymes (Whipple *et al.,* 1990; de Lisle *et al.,* 1992 and Baufriend *et al.* 1996). Recently Patel *et al.* (2006) sequenced K-10 genome of *Mycobacterium avium* subspp. *paratuberculosis* (Map) by means of RNA isolation and DNA microarry as well as RT-PCR.

Serological Approaches for detection of Map infection

In the infected individual, the level of humoral infection is related with fecal shedding of the organisms. In early stage of infection strong cell mediated immune response elicited which leads to a delay type hypersensitivity reaction, but when the disease in progress gradually CMI become fleeted and there is welcoming of a strong humoral immune response and at the edge of final stage due to lack of antigen specific CMI, there is rapid dissemination of infection throughout the host (Benedixen, 1978). The AGID (Agar Gel Immunodiffusion) assay is an inexpensive mode of serological diagnosis in ruminants paratuberculosis, which can detect antibody within 3-9 months after sheeding of microbes (Colgrove *et al.,* 1989). As the specificity of the test is 100% so it is a reliable test to detect Map. Another serological reliable test to detect Map. is ELISA (Enzyme Linked Immuno sorbent Assay), which is superior than AGID as it has both high sensitivity the test is 100% so it is a and specificity. Numerous modified techniques of PCR are available for detection of *M. paratuberculosis* infection. To reduces the chance of cross contamination it is necessary to characterised and isolate *M. paratuberculosis* species specific antigens. In the terminal stages due to immuneanargy sensitivity of serological tests may be very low as 10 to 25% only (Coussens, 2001).

Cell mediated immunity based diagnosis

CMI assay invovled DTH assay; lymphocyte stimulating assay and gama interferon assay. As we have already cited that CMI response only present in early stage of infection so these above mention tests are negative during advance stage of infection. Skin test using johnin is not so reliable. This test is performed by intradermal inoculation of Map extract (johnin). An increase in the thickness of skin at the site of inoculation (4 mm or more) within 72 hours is consider as positive. This test is less sensitive(54%) as well as less sensitive(79%), also has poor correlation with the infectious status of animals (Hremel *et al.,* 1998).

Gamma interferon are better indicator of CMI assay for both research and diagnostic purposes, which released by peripheral blood mononuclear cell in response to antigen is estimated by ELISA using monoclonal antibody against gamma interferons. Two assays known as a bioassay (Wood *et al.,* 1989) and sandwich enzyme immuneassay(SEIA) have been evaluated (Rothel *et al.,* 1990). But some results indicated that this test is not so specific and reliable for diagnosis of paratuberculosis infection (Mc Donald *et al.,* 1999 and Ridge *et al.,* 1995).

Humoral immunity based diagnostic methods

AGID has a high specificity(>90%) in animals with clinical signs but due to lower sensitivity (30%), this test is not reliable for diagnostic purposes(Wood *et al.,* 1989).

Next of AGID is complement fixation test or CFT . The specificity of thi test is less than AGID and ELISA. This test can detects antibodies 1-5 months later than ELISA (Singh *et al.,* 2005) and it has intermediate sensitivity to AGID and ELISA. So CFT is not used in routine diagnostic tests.

ELISA is one of the most valuable herd screening test for detection of paratuberculosis. Although the sensitivioty of this test is higher in clinically infected animals but low at initial and terminal stages of disease. It was showed that ELISA sensitivity for clinical and subclinical cases are 85% and 15% respectively (Wood *et al.,* 1989). An indigenous ELISA by using protoplasmic antigen from Native "Bison type"strain of Map has been developed for screening of paratuberculosis infection in animals aswellas humans (Singh *et al.,*2007). ELISA can be used for 'herd screening test' also. Pre absorption of sera with M.Pheli is a good candidate to increase assay specificity but reduces the sensitivity. It was reported that only 1/3 rd of animals shedding Map can be detected by present ELISA tests (Collins *et al.,* 1989). So it is very much essential to search for Map specific antigens and to characterized them for sero diagnostic purposes.

Recombinant antigens for detection of anti M.A. paratuberculosis antibodies

A large scale postgenomic analysis of Map proteins identified various specific antigens that could potentially improve the diagnosis of paratuberculosis. Cho *et al.,* (2007) identified fourteen proteins of potential diagnostic value for bovine paratuberculosis. These proteins were ultimately designed by mass spectroscopy and BLAST analysis as ModD, PepA , ArgJ, CobT, Antigen 85c and nine hypothetical proteins. These 14 antigenic proteins from *M.A. paratuberculosis* culture filtrate (CF) are a good candidates for use as antigens for improvement of serodiagnostic tests for bovine paratuberculosis .Screening of genomic expression library with serum of naturally infected cattle, Willemsen and his colleagues have identified and characterized three novel secreted *M.a. paratuberculosis* antigens of 9, 15 and 34 kDa sizes(Willemsen *et al.,* 2006). An absorption ELISA based diagnostic test using 34 kDa protein was established which having high specificity and sensitivity and can be useful for screening of johne's disease(Malamo *et al.,* 2006). Carboxy terminal end of this 34 Kda protein is 100% specific for Map (Ostrowski M *et al.,* 2003). Two secretary proteins Ahp C and Ahp D having the ability to differentiate paratuberculosis and tuberculosis (Tizard M L V *et al.,* 1992).Antibodies at higher level against a 14 kDa secreted antigen were detected in patients with crhon's disese (Shin S J *et al.,* 2004).

Recently a highly specific and sensitive Ethanol Vortex ELISA(EV ELISA) was developed for diagnosis of paratuberculosis by using antigens extracted from surface of the organism. Study has shown that EV ELISA is subspecies specific and highly sensitive to detect early aswell as late state of *M.A. paratuberculosis* infections (Eda *et al.,* 2006).

Lpp34 is an unique membrane protein of Map , which is a putative lipoprotein (Gioffre *etal* 2006). Lipoprotein have long been considered immunomodulators and mycobacteria are especially rich in these post translationally modified proteins. As Lpp 34 is an envelop protein of the bacteria, so it can perform a numerous and important functions including adhesion to host tissues, nutrient acquistation and interection with host defences. These Lpp 34 can be used to identify specific antibody of *M.A. paratuberculosis.*

A 35 kDa protein of M.A. Paratuberculosis was studied for its ability to elicit CMI response using mouse model (Basagoudanavar *et al.,* 2006). So, a 35kDa protein can be used as a diagnostic test to measure delay type hypersensitivity response in paratuberculosis infection. It was also suggested that a 35 kDa based ELISA can be useful for detecting *M.a. paratuberculosis* infection (Sung *et al.*,2005).

A 19 kDa lipoprotein was identified which can stimulate both T and B cell immune responses as well as induce a number Th1 cytokines.In order to evaluate the *M.A. Paratuberculosis* 19 kDa lipoprotein can act as immune modulator in cattle with johne's disease and has been shown to stimulate CD4+ Tcell proliferation as well asrelase of IL-2,IFN-γ and IL-2. Acylation near the N terminal portion of the 19 kDa protein is believed to occur at amino acids 19-24 and contributes to it's immunogenecity. Further more glycosylation of the *M.paratuberculosis* 19 kDa protein inhibits innate immune response , such as releaseof TNFalpha, IL-6 and IL-10 from macrophages,but doesnot affect antibody bindings. Huntley and his groups demonstrated that this 19 kDa protein can be used to assess cellular immune responses in subclinically infected cattle as well as humoral immune responses in cattle with clinical johen's disease (Huntley *etal.*,2005).

A lipoarabinomanan(LAM) antigen which was extracted from the lymphnode and milk of partuberculosis infected sheep and goat ,can be used to raised antibody and thus can be useful for serodiagnostic tests (Munjal etal., 2004).

An exported 22 kDa putative lipoprotein was identified in an alkaline phosphatase gene fusion library of *Mycobacterium avium paratuberculosis* and expressed in *Mycobacterium smegmatis* to produce a C-terminal polyhistidin-tagged protein, which can elicit interferon gamma secretion in blood of vaccinated animals (Rigden *et al.,* 2006)

With complete genome sequencing of Map K10 post genomic application will play a central role for detection of Map specific antigens and some has already done in this horizon. Results of comparative genomics and proteomics assay of Map culture extracts, 25 Map diagnostic antigens were identified (Bannantine and Paustian , 2006). In silico comparision of Map genome with other mycobacterial genomes and cloning aswell asexpression of Map unique protein sequences Map specific protein antigens were identified that reacted with sera from infected animals (Cho and Collins , 2006).Genome sequencing of Map K10 had identified 3 Map unique IS elements IS Map 2, Map 02 Map 04 present in 3, 4, 6 copies respectively. Comparative genomics based study identified 17 Map unique large sequence polymorphism (LSPs) (Stevenson *et al.*, 2002).

Conclusion and future perspectives

With the critical need for improved diagnostic tests to detect paratuberculosis infection, effort need to be concentrated on the development of simple, rapid, noninvasive tests that can perform without expensive laboratory equipment. In this situation search for a novel antigen candidate suitable for specific and sensitive diagnosis and/or vaccination appears to be a well justified approach and need for the hour.

References

Bannantine J P& Paustain M L, (2006) *Methods Mol Biol*, **345**:185

Bannantine, J.P., Hansen, J.K., Paustian, M.L., Amonsin, A., Li, L.L., Stabel, J.R. and Kapur, V. (2004). . *Am. Societ. Microbiol.,* 42: 106-114

Basagoudanavar, S.H., Goswami, P.P. and Tiwari, V. (2006). *Vet. Res. Commun.,***30**: 357-367.

Baufreind R, Benazzi S, Weiss R, Schliesser T, Williems H, baljer G. (1996). *J. Clinical Microbiology*. 1617-1621.

Benedixen P. H. (1978). *Nord. Vety. Medicine*. **30:** 163-1621.

Chiodini, R.J., Van Kruiningen,H.J., Merkal,R.S.(1984). *Cornell Vet.,***74**, 218-262.

Cho D , Shin S J, Talaat A M. & Collins M T., (2007) *Expr Purif, **PMID*** : 17296312 (in press).

Cho D& Collins M T,(2006) *Clin Vacc Immunol*,**13:**1155

Colgrove, G.F., C.O. Thoen, B.O. Blackburn and C.D. Murphy (1989).*Vety. Microbiology,* **19:** 183-187.

Collins, M.T. (1996). *Vet. Clin. N. Am. Food. Anim. Prac.,* **12**: 357 371.

Coussens, P.M. (2001). *Animal Health Res. Rev.,***2**: 141-161.

de Lisle, G.W., Collins, D.M., Huchzermeyer, H.F.A.K. (1992). *Onder J. Vet. Res.,* **59:** 163-165.

Eda S., Bannantine JP, Waters W R, Mori Y, Whitlock RH, Scott MC & Speer C A., (2006) *lin Vaccine Immunol.* **13(8)**: 837-44

Ghadiali AH, Strother M, Naser SA, Manning EJB & Sreevatsan S (2004) *J.Clin.Microbiol***42**: 5345-5348

Gioffre A, Caimi K, Zumarraga M J, Meikle V, Morsella C, Bigi F, Alito A, Santangelo M P, Paolicchi F., Romano M I & Cataldi A (2006) *J Vet Med B Infect Dis Vet Public Health*. **53(1):** 34-41

Grant, I.R., Ball, H.J. and Rowe, M.R. (1999). *Lett. Appl. Microbiol.,* **28**: 461-465.

Harris, N.B. and Barletta, R.G. (2001). *Clin. Microbiol. Rev.***14**: 489-512.

Hawkey, P.M. (1994). *Reviews of Medical Microbiology***5:** 21-23.

Hermel S R, (1998).*Angus .J.,***3:**194

Hughes, B.M., Stevenson, K. and Sharp, J.M. (2000). *J. Microbiological Methods,* **44:** 209-215.

Huntley, J.F., Stabel, J.R., Paustian, M.L., Reinhardt, T.A. and Bannantine, J.P. (2005). *Infect. Immun.,***73**: 6877-6884

Kunze, Z. M., Portaels, F., and McFadden, J. J., (1992). *J. Clinic. Microbiol.,***30**: 2366-2372.

Malamo M., Sakoda Y., Ozaki H & Kida H., (2006) *Jpn J Vet Res* ,**54**: 99

Mc Donald W L, Ridge S E, Hope A F & Condron R J. (1999) *Aus. Vet J* ,**77** : 113

MotiwalaAS, Amonsin A, Strother M, Manning EJB,Kapur V & Sreevatsan S (2004) *J.Clin. Microbiol* **42**: 1703-1712

Munjal S K., Boehmer J., Beyerbach M., Strutzberg-Minder K., Homuth M.(2004) *Vet.Microbiol*.**103 (1-2):** 107-14

Naser, S.A., Ghobrial, G., Romero, C. and Valentine, J.F. (2004). *Lancet,***364**: 1039-1044

Ostrowski M., Mundo SL, Harris N B, Barletta R G & Lopez O J.,(2003) *Scand J Immunol,* **58** : 511

Patel D, Lia Danelishbili, Yoshitka Yamazki, Marta Alonso Michael L. Paustian, John P. Bannantine, Lisbeth Meunier-Goddik and Luiz E. Bermudez (2006): *Infect. and Immun.* **74** : 2849-2855

Ridges S E, Harkin JT, Badman R T, Mellor A M & Larsen J W ,(1995) *Aus. Vet J,* **72**: 150

Rigden R C., Jandhyala D M ., Dupnot C, Crosbie-Caird D., Lopez-Villalobos N, Maeda N., Gicqel B, Murray A.(2006) *J Med Microbiol,* **55**: 1735-40

Rothel J.S, Jones S L., Corner L A., Cox J C & Wood P R, A. (1990) . *Aust Vet J,* **67** 134

Shin S J., Yoo H S., Mc Donough S P & Chang Y F,(2004) . *J Vet Sci,* **5:** 111

Singh A V, Singh SV & Gupta V. K.(2005) *International Association for Paratuberculosis, Denmark.* 344

Singh S V, Singh AV ,Singh P.K., Gupta V K, Kumar S., & Vohra J., (2007). *Small Ruminant Research.***70**: 89-92

Stevenson, K. and Sharp,J.M. (1997). *The Vety. Journal,* **153:** 269-286.

Stevenson, K., Hughes, V.M., de Juan, L., Inglis,N.F., Wright, F. and Sharp, J.M.(2002). *J.Clin. Microbiol.***40:** 1798-1804 .

Stvenson K., Hughes V M., de Juan L., Inglis, D F., Wright F&Sharp J M., (2002) *J Clin Microbiol,***40:**1798

Sung Jae Shin, Chao-Fu Chang ,Ching-Dong Chang, Sean P., Mc Donough, Belinda Thompson , Han Sang Yoo & Yung-Fu Chang (2005) *Infection and Immunity,* **73(8)** 5074-85

Thorel, M.F., Krichevsky, M. and Levy, V.V. (1990). *Int. J. Syst. Bacteriol.,***40**: 254-260.

Tizard M L V, Moss M T., Sanderson J D., Austen B M. & Hermon- Taylor J,(1992). *J Gen Microbiol,* **138:** 1728

Twort, F.W. and G.L.Y. Ingram. (1912). *Proc.Soc.London.*,**99**: 1323-1329.

Wells S.J. and Wagner, B.A. (2000). *J. Amer. Vet. Med. Associat.*,**216**, 1450–1457.

Whipple D.L. Karpe and Vary c.(1990). *J.clinical Microbiology*.**28**:2561-2564

Whipple D.L. Karpe and Vary C.(1990).*J clinical Microbiology*.**28**:2561-2564

Willemsen P T, Westerveen J, Dinkla A, Bakker D, Van Zijderveld FG & Thole J E., (2006) *Vet Microbiol*, **114**: 337

Wood P R, Kopsidas K., Milner A R., Hill J,Gilll., Webb R., Mack W N. & Coates K. (1989). *CSRIOPublications,Melbourne, Australia*, 164.

□□□

Chapter 10

Candidate Gene based Approach for Mastitis Resistance Breeding

UMESH SINGH, RAJIB DEB, SUSHIL KUMAR AND ARJAVA SHARMA
Project Directorate on Cattle, ICAR, Meerut-250 001, UP, India

Mastitis is an inflammatory reaction of the mammarygland, usually to a microbial infection, and its prevalenceis alarming. Mastitis is characterized by an influx of somatic cells,primarily polymorphonuclear neutrophils (PMN), intothemammary gland and by an increase in milk proteasecontent. Clinical infections are diagnosedby red, swollen appearance of the gland andflakes or clots (protein aggregates) in the milk. Subclinicalinfections, by definition, show no obvious signs of disease.

Etiology

Five bacterial species namely *Staphylococcus aureus,Streptococcus dysgalactiae, Streptococcus agalactiae,Streptococcus uberis,* and *Escherichia coli*are responsiblefor the bulk of bovine mastitis cases. *Staphylococcus aureus, S. dysgalactiae,* and *S. agalactiae* exhibita contagious route of transmission, whereas *S. uberis*and *E. coli* are considered to be environmental agents. Yeast can also cause mastitis. Overuse of antibiotics and poor sanitation contribute toyeast mastitis.

Symptoms

1. Inflammation is characterized by Gross abnormalities in the udder (swelling, heat, redness, pain).

2. Persisting inflammation leads to tissue damage and replacement of secretory tissues with of the udder with nonproductive connective tissues.
3. Change in composition (Table 1) and appearance of milk.
4. Abnormalities in milk may include flakes, clots or a watery appearance. The flakes in the milk are congealed leukocytes, secretory cells and protein.
5. A lower milk yield.

Pathogenesis

Mastitis begins after bacteria pass through the teat duct and enter the cisternal area. Invasion of the teat usually occurs during milking. Organisms present in the milk or at the teat end enter the teat canal and cistern when there is admission of undesired air in the milking unit. After milking, the teat canal remains dilated for 1-2 hours while the canal of a damaged teat may remain partially open permanently. This makes it easier for organisms from the environment or those found on injured skin to enter the teat canal. Adherenceof bacteria to tissues lining cisterns and ducts may prevent flushing-out during milking and help establish infections. Bacteria eventually enter the glandular tissues where they affect alveolar cells. Toxins produced by bacteria cause death of or damage to milk-secreting epithelial cells, and these cells produce substances to the blood stream that increase blood vessel permeability. This allows leukocytes to move from the blood into the alveolus where they function by engulfing bacteria.

Types of Mastitis

There are several ways of classifying mastitis. A simple classification recognize mastitis as two major groups:

A *Contagious Mastitis*: Caused by bacteria live on the skin of the teat and inside the udder. Contagious mastitis can be transmitted from one cow to another during milking.

B *Environmental mastitis*: Describes mastitis caused by organisms such as *Escherichia coli* which do not normally live on the skin or in the udder but which enter the teat canalwhen the cow comes in contact with a contaminated environment. The pathogens normally found in feces bedding materials, and feed. Cases of environmental mastitisrarely exceed 10% of the total mastitis cases in the herd.

Contagious mastitis can be divided into three groups:

1. Clinical mastitis
2. Sub-clinical mastitis
3. Chronic mastitis

Table 1 : Changes in milk composition associated with mastitis.

Composition	Normal milk	Mastitis Milk
Solid non fat	8.98	8 99
Fat	35	3.20
Lactose	4.90	4.40
Total protein	3.61	3.56
Casein	2.82	2.30
Whey	0.81	1.30
Serum albumine	0.02	0.07
Lactoferrin	0.02	0.10
Immunoglobulins	0.10	0.60
Sodium	0.06	0.10
Cholride	0.09	0.14
Potassium	0.17	0.15
Calcium	0.12	0.04

1. Clinical mastitis

Characterized by the presence of gross inflammation signs (swelling, heat, redness, pains). Three types of clinical mastitis exist. *Peracute mastitis* Characterized by gross inflammation, disrupted functions (reduction in milk yield,changes in milk composition) and systemic signs (fever, depression, shivering, loss ofappetite and loss of weight), *Acute mastitis* Similar to percute mastitis, but with lesser systemic signs (fever and mild depression).*and Sub-acute mastitis* In this type of mastitis, the mammary gland inflammation signs are minimal and novisible systemic signs.

2. Sub-clinical mastitis

This form of mastitis is characterized by change in milk composition with no signs of gross inflammation or milk abnormalities. Changes in milk composition can be detected by special diagnostic tests.The vast majority of mastitis are "subclinical". The number of somatic cells in the milk, an indicative of the inflammatory response, may be elevated and bacterial can be cultured from the milk.

3. Chronic mastitis

An inflammatory process that exists for months, and may continue from one lactation to another. Chronic mastitis for the most part exist as sub-clinical but may exhibit periodical flare-ups sub-acute or acute form, which last for a short period of time.

Somatic Cell Count (SCC)

Somatic cells are normal constituent of milk and only when they become excessive do they indicate a problem. Somatic cells are composed of leucocytes (75%) and epithelial cells (25%). Leucocytes (white blood cells) increase in milk in response to infection or injury while increase in epithelial cells is the result of infection or injury. The number of cells reflects the severity of mastitis. Somatic cells are expressed either as cells/ml of milk (Somatic Cell Count, SCC) or as Somatic Cell Score (SCS).The SCC of "normal" milk is less than 200,000 cells/ml. Higher counts are considered abnormal and indicate possible infections. To be used for human consumption, milk must have less than 750,000 SCC. Milk markets rely routinely on SCC to help ensure good quality milk and usually pay a premium for milk with low SCC. This is because high SCC causes a rise in whey protein and a decrease in casein resulting in a considerable lower cheese yields. A shorter shelf life and adverse milk flavors are other consequences of high SCC. Higher counts are also associated with decreased production. When individual cows have a SCC between 250,000-300,000 (SCS = 4) that usually indicates a subclinical mastitiscaused by major pathogens. Somatic cell counts can be conducted on individual cows or on bulk tank samples (Bulk Tank Somatic Cell Counts, BTSCC). If conducted accurately, BTSCC can provide a general indication of a herd's mastitis status. Although BTSCC may be a good indicator of the herd's udder health status, it will not identify problem cows nor locate factors contributing to their high counts. Although BTSCC may be a good indicator of the herd's udder health status, it will not identify problem cows nor locate factors contributing to their high counts. Somatic cell counts on composite milk samples for each cow are usually available for herds on Dairy Herd Improvement (DHI). Electronic cell counting instruments estimate milk SCC from the same sample that is used for testing fat and protein.

Diagnosis of Mastitis

The first step in treating mastitis is to identify the causative agent. The presence of a pathogen and the inflammatory response of the udder signify an infection. The inflammatory response, which results in abnormal milk is usually detected by the dairyman.Because mastitis is frequently subclinical "hidden", a number of tests have been developed for detecting mastitis. Most tests estimate the Somatic Cell Counts (SCC) of a milk sample. There is no one somatic cell count at which a cow is free from mastitis. A level of 50,000 cell/ml of milk is usually used as a beginning point for closer observation. A variety of tests are available to determine the presence or absence of clinical and subclinical mastitis. The majority of these tests primarily indicate inflammation in the udder. They do not measure infection or bacterial presence.

The Stripcup Test

The stripcup or strip plate is an important in the milking parlor for determining the presence of clinical mastitis. The test is rapid and can easily be adapted as a part of milking routine. Few streams of the foremilk are squirted onto the strip cup and are visually examined for milk abnormalities. The stripcup test should be conducted on every cow at every milking and milk from any cow found to have abnormal milk should be withhold from the supply. In addition to the identification of clinical mastitis, the use of the stripcup has other benefits. The stripping of the first streams of milk stimulates milk let-down, resulting in a faster milk out which can result in a shorter milking time. Removal of the foremilk may reduce bacterialcontamination of the milking machine and thus reduce the probability of udder contamination and enhance the quality of milk produced.

The California Mastitis Test (CMS)

The CMT estimates the number somatic cells present in the milk. The CMT is conducted by mixing the test reagent with an equal quantity of milk. It reacts with materials from the nuclei of the somatic cells in the milk to form a gel. The reaction is then visually scored depending on the amount of gel formedThe CMT is a simple, inexpensive, rapid screening test and is useful in determining which quarter of the cow is most affected. However, the CMT can not be used as a means of picking out cows for treatments as it all detects is a cellular response to inflammation. The test is useful in indicating sub-clinical and chronic mastitis.

Wisconsin Mastitis Test

This is a laboratory test that is generally conducted on bulk tank samples. The test uses the same reagent as the CMT. However, the reaction is not estimated but measured and thus the WMT is more precise than the CMT. The WMT results are generally reported in mm. However, the scores can be used to predict the average number of somatic cells.The test is usually used as a screening test on producer's milk due to its simplicity and objectivity. Samples score higher than 19 mm are subjected to further tests and scrutiny. The test also provides a convenient method of monitoring udder health on a herd basis by examining the cows, milking equipment, milking procedure and outside environment when WMT values starts to increase.Based on the WMT, the goal for the herd should be to maintain a bulk tan reading of less than 8 mm (300,000 cells/ml). Milk with a WMT score of 19 mm (855,000) or greater is generally considered unsuitable for human consumption

Electronic Somatic Cell Count

This an automated and centralized system for somatic cell count which is used by Dairy Herd Improvement Associations. The procedure is more precise than the CMT and the WMT. The main disadvantages are that the equipment is expensive and requires constant monitoring. The test can be used to monitor the udder health of individual cows as well as the udder health of the entire herd.

Control of Mastitis

Prevention is the key in mastitis control. A control program should emphasize factors that reduce the rate of new infections. A combination of preventive measures and therapeutic use ofantibiotics will markedly reduce the incidence of mastitis.

The prevention of mastitis can be achieved by:

Proper milking hygiene : Bacteria transmit to the uninfected from the contaminated hands of the milker. Thus the milker's hands should be washed thoroughly with disinfected soaps before milking and clinically infected cows should be milked last. Teats should be cleaned and dried before milking.

Milking machine : Should function and operate properly. Vacuum level in the milkingunit should be between 275 and 300 mm of mercury with little fluctuation. The vacuum regulator should be kept clean and checked regularly.

Dipping the teats after milking : Teat dipping does not reduce existing infection. However, the rate of new infection can be reduced by up to 50% when suitable disinfectant is used to immerse or spry the teats.

Dry treatments : Incidence of mastitis during the dry period can be considerably reduced by effective use of antibiotic infused in each quarter of the udder at the last milking of a lactation. Dry cow therapy is the best way to cure chronic and subclinical mastitis that are difficult to treat successfully during lactation.

Culling of chronically infected cows : This is an effective method because in most herds only 6-8% of all cows account for 40-50% of all clinical mastitis.

Nutrition : Deficiencies of selenium and vitamin E in the diet have been associated with an increased rate of new mammary infections.

Treatment of Mastitis

The decision to treat all cows at drying off in contrast to treating selected cows during lactation is influenced by type of organism causing the mastitis and the extent of the problem in the herd. Acute mastitis such as that caused by coliform bacteria endangers the cow's life and requires immediate attention of a veterinarian. Milking the affected quarter every 2-3 hours helps to eliminate toxins. Treatment of clinical mastitis limits the duration and possible spread of the disease. When an antibiotic treatment is recommended, it is very critical to follow instruction, especially regarding the duration of treatment. Only mastitis caused by *S. agalactiae* can be treated successfully with antibiotics during lactation. The success rate of antibiotics in treating mastitis cause by *S. aureus* and coliform bacteria does not exceed 50% could be as low as 10%). Subclinical mastitis (high SCC in milk) should not be treated with antibiotics during lactation and they are treated at the time of drying off.

Transgenic Approach to Enhance Mastitis Resistance

The use of transgenesis to direct expression of a foreign protein into mouse milk was first reported in 1987.Shortly thereafter, it was proposed that mammary production of trout lysozyme II or bacterial lysostaphin would be an effective means to enhance mastitis resistance. Both of these proteins have considerable antistaphylococcal activity. However, the initial applications of the technology were the generation of transgenic mice producing human lysozyme or human lactoferrin in milk. Milk from various lines of the lysozyme-transgenic mice contained approximately 0.5 mg/ml of human lysozyme. Bioactivity of the lysozyme, as detected by its ability to degrade *Micrococcus lysodeikticus* cell walls, was retained. Limited, but significant bacteriostatic activity of the milk against *S.aureus*, but not a mastitis-causing clinical isolate of *E.coli*, was also found . Further, the lysozyme-containing milk also slowed the growth of the cold spoilage organisms *Pseudomonas fragi* and *Lactobacillusviscous*, indicating the potential of this strategy to also address issues of product shelf life and food safety.

Transgenic technology has resulted in the production of mice and cows that secrete human lactoferrin into their milk . Lactoferrin is an iron-binding glycoprotein found in most exocrine secretions including tears, saliva, and milk, and there are numerous reports of its antibacterial activity in vitro and in vivo. Although bovine milk normally contains low levels of lactoferrin, the transgenic cows were generated as potential bioreactors to produce large quantities of recombinant hLF (rhLF) for applications in human health care. The mechanism of lactoferrin activity has not been clearly defined but appears to stem primarily through iron sequestration or through direct interaction of its cationic *N*-terminal region with bacterial components. The contribution of bLF to protection of the mammary gland is compromised by its low concentration in milk and the presence of other milk constituents. Thus, milk citrate can effectively compete with lactoferrin for iron binding and the resulting iron-citrate complex can be utilized by bacteria.

Defensins are another class of antibacterial protein that are produced in neutrophils, macrophages, and epithelial cells lining mucosal surfaces .Their antibacterial action appears to result from their ability to form pores in target membranes leading to cell lysis. Analogous antibacterial peptides have been isolated from a diverse array of multicellular organisms including insects, amphibians, and plants and are currently being evaluated as topical antibiotics for human medicine. Transgenic mice have been generated that produce small quantities (5 μg/ml) of a mammalian defensin—bovine tracheal antimicrobial peptide (**bTAP**)—in their milk. The bTAP purified from milk was bioactive in vitro, but no challenge studies were reported. Transgenic mice that secrete lysostaphin into their milk provide a clear demonstration of the transgenic approach to enhancing mastitis resistance. Lysostaphin is a potent peptidoglycan hydrolase naturally secreted by *Staphylococus simulans*.

Another transgenic approach to enhance disease resistance involves the production of pathogen-specificantibodies into milk . To date, the primary goal ofthese projects has been to supply antibodies to offspringand thus provide enhanced passive immunity. However,with these projects as proof of concept it is notinconceivable that antibodies to mastitis causing pathogenscould enhance protection of the mammary gland.Two of the reports indicate the potential of producingcoronavirus neutralizing antibodies into milk under thecontrol of the 5'-regulatory regions of the murine whey acidic protein (WAP) gene or theoBLG gene. In both instancestransgenic mice secreted functional antibody into milkas determined by an in vitro neutralization assay.

Candidate Antibacterial Proteins for Mastitis Resistance

One of the protein called lysostaphin that are able to cleave the peptidoglycan of the bacterial cell wall. The peptidoglycan is the structural framework of the cell wall, and its degradation exposes the bacteria to mechanical damage, and osmotic lysis. The transgenic animal strategy opens the doorto utilization of these nonmammalian enzymes withthe possibility that a combination of enzymes may beeffective against all species of mastitis pathogens, andthat the combination approach against any particular species may limit the development of resistant bacteria.

Bacteriophage lysis is generally mediated by the production of two proteins, a holin and a lysin. The holin creates a hole in the cell membrane that enables the lysin to access the peptidoglycan. Thelysin then degrades the peptidoglycan resulting in lysis of the bacteria. This phenomenon is known as "lysis from within," and in contrast, external addition of the lysin to a gram-negative bacteria such as *E. coli* does not result in lysis presumably because the lysin can not access the peptidoglycan through the outer cell membrane. However, the application of phage lysins to treat infections caused by gram-positive bacteria, which lack an outer membrane, is seeing a resurgence. Recently, streptococcal phage lysins have been shown to be very effective in the treatment of experimentally induced nasopharyngeal, streptococcal infections.

Candidate Gene Regulatory Regions

The production of novel proteins into milk of transgenic animals has relied on the incorporation of milk protein regulatory regions into the transgene constructs. This ensures production of the protein in lactating mammary epithelium. However, mastitis susceptibility is not confined to the lactating state. In fact, transition periods, either from the dry to lactating state or vice versa, are periods of enhanced susceptibility to mastitis. This has led us to explore genes known to be active in these states as candidate regulatory regionsfor a transgenic approach to enhance mastitis resistance.

Disease resistant genes for mastitis

The mammary gland is typically a sterile environment and, therefore, the entry of any foreign body usually triggers a localized immune response. The first line of defence against disease-causing microorganisms is the innate immune system, which induces mechanisms that are not pathogen species-specific . Innate immune cells in the mammary gland are comprised of macrophages, granulocytes, natural killer cells, and dendritic and mammary epithelial cells . These cells have receptors that recognize motifs or pathogen-associated molecular patterns (PAMP) on the surface of microorganisms. For example, the lipopolysaccharides on the surface of Gram-negative bacteria such as E. coli become attached to the phagocytic cells via Toll-like receptor 4 (TLR-4), whereas Toll-like receptor 2 (TLR-2) binds to Gram-positive motifs such aspeptidoglycan or lipoteichoic acid on the surface of S.aureus. Recognition of an invading pathogen activates cellular reactions, leading to the secretion of inflammatory mediators called cytokines. These signalling molecules trigger cellular communication, chemotaxis and lymphocyte differentiation. The cytokines include inflammatory interleukins-(IL)-1β, -6 and -12, tumour necrosis factor-alpha (TNF-α) and interferon-gamma (IFN-γ) . Once phagocytic cells recognize and internalize pathogens, the cells present the pathogen's antigenic determinants to the T lymphocytes. Then these cells, in the presence of IL-12, differentiate into Th1 effector cells which are responsible for cell-mediated immunity. These Th1 cells produce inflammatory mediators such as IFN-γ, that enhance macrophage effectors functions against intracellular pathogens. Macrophages are the predominant cells in the healthy mammary gland . During intramammary infection however, a release of inflammatory mediators, especially by macrophages, leads to the recruitment of neutrophils into infected quarters from the circulation. At this stage, these cells account for more than 90% of milk cells . The neutrophils are responsible for the eventual elimination of the pathogens. For example, activated neutrophils degranulate and produce/secrete bactericidal components, namely reactive oxygen species (ROS) . The recruitment of neutrophils into the mammary gland causes an increase in somatic cell count (SCC) that can reach more than 1,000,000 cells/mL during the course of an infection, whereas the SCC is normally less than 100,000 cells/mL in a healthy mammary gland. Prevention and control of mastitis by improving the natural defence mechanisms is important not only for dairy producers but also for consumers, because of increased concerns about food safety, antibiotic use and animal welfare. One approach would be to define breeding objectives with increased weight of health-related traits in genetic selection . Genetic selection to increase antibody responsiveness seems to be possible, but the acquired immune response traits have proven to be inconsistent indicators of udder health . Components of the adaptive immune system have been studied intensively, but there is still need for the development of efficient vaccine against pathogens that cause intramammary infection for bovine . Unlike the adaptive immune system, some mechanisms of the innate immunity are conserved throughout the animal kingdom and can thus be thought of as general mechanisms responsible for broad environmental responses. These evolutionarily conserved systems have been analyzed in detail and include, among others, the complement gene family and the Toll-like receptors (TLR) . The parameters of innate immune responses can be used to study resistance to mastitis. These results can lead to the selection of breeding animals that carry favorable polymorphisms or alleles able to improve the resistance.

A fair amount of genetic research related to lactation and udder health has already been performed due to its economic importance for milk production and manufacturing. This has led to considerable improvement of milk yield (MY); however, the progress in technological properties of milk and udder health has been relatively slow.to infection of their offspring. It has been reported that somatic cell score (SCS) associated loci have been proposed to improve resistance to mastitis in dairy cattle. Most estimates of the genetic correlation between SCS and clinical mastitis range from 0.50 to 0.80. The SCC distribution is often highly skewed and it is usually transformed on a logarithm scale, as follows: SCS = log2 (SCC/100,000) + 3. When used for genetic evaluation, bulls receive an estimated breeding value (EBV) based on the SCS records of their daughters. If dairy producers select bulls with a low EBV for SCS, this is expected to improve mastitis resistance in their herd . The SCS has now become the most important indicator associated with the health of the mammary gland, but little is known about the key factors which regulate the number of somatic cells in milk from healthy cows. Thus, some of the studies undertaken to investigate the early activated transcripts of immune cells of the lactating mammary gland in order to identify key genes in the innate immune response to mastitis. In addition, the expression of micro RNAs (miRNAs) in the bovine mammary gland could also play an important role in regulatory path-ways in mammary gland development, milk production and resistance or susceptibility to mastitis (Silveri *et al.* 2006). Functional traits of the mammary gland have been studied using different approaches, including the QTL approach, association studies and the candidate gene approach.One of the candidate gene related to mastitis resistant, discovered was osteopontin (or secreted phosphoprotein 1, SPP1). Osteopontin is a cytokine produced by macrophages and activated T cells. Osteopontin has been described as an early component of the T cell activation mechanism. Enhanced in T cells, it recruits macrophages at the infection site and improves cell-mediated immunity (Th1) by inducing secretion of Th1 cytokines. Osteopontin is a multi-faced protein. It promotes bone remodelling, wound healing and survival of stressed cells, but is also associated with metastasis status and poor survival prognosis . It was found associated with certain pathologies such as restenosis, formation of kidney stones, and autoimmune disease , but also found to confer resistance to several intracellular pathogen infections through recruitment and activation of macrophages. This study reported that the link between DNA polymorphisms of SPP1, the number of milk immune cells and, potentially, the susceptibility to mastitis. These SNPs were identified by in silico search to be located in transcription factor recognition sites which factors are presumably involved in the Th1 immune response and in the Th2 regulation pathway. Indeed, one SNP abolished the SP1 recognition site, whereas another SNP affected the transcription binding factor mIKAROS. All together, these findings support the genetic potential of these variants in terms of selection for the improvement of mastitis resistance in dairy cows.

References

Alain K., Karrow N.A., Thibault C., St-Pierre J., Lessard M,. Bissonnette N..2009. Osteopontin: an early innate immune marker of Escherichia coli mastitis harbors genetic polymorphisms with possible links with resistance to mastitis. BMC Genomics. 18; 10:444.

Auldist, M. J., S. Coats, G. L. Rogers, and G. H. McDowell. 1995.Changes in the composition of milk from healthy and mastiticdairy cows during the lactation cycle. Aust. J. Exp. Agricul.35:427–436.

Auldist, M. J., S. J. Coats, B. J. Sutherland, J. F. Hardham, G. H.McDowell, and G. L. Rogers. 1996. Effect of somatic cell countand stage of lactation on the quality and storage life of ultrahigh temperature milk. J. Dairy Res. 63:377–386.

Bar D., Tauer L.W., Bennett G, González R.N., Hertl J.A., Schukken Y.H., Schulte H.F., Welcome F.., Gröhn Y.T.2008.The cost of generic clinical mastitis in dairy cows as estimated by using dynamic programming. J. Dairy Sci. 91(6):2205-2214.

Barbano, D. M., R. R. Rasmussen, and J. M. Lynch. 1991. Influenceof milk somatic cell count and milk age on cheese yield. J. DairySci. 74: 369–388.

Barkema, H.W. 1998. Incidence of clinical mastitis in dairy herds grouped in three categories by bulk milk somatic cell counts . J Dairy Sci, 812, 411–419.

Bayles, K. W., C. A. Wesson, L. E. Liou, L. K. Fox, G. A. Bohach,and W. R. Trumble. 1998. Intracellular Staphylococcus aureusescapes the endosome and induces apoptosis in epithelial cells.Infect. Immun. 66:336–342.

Berry, D. P., Bermingham, M.L., Good, M. and More,S.J.2011. Genetics of animal health and disease in cattle Veterinary Journal 64:5.

Bramley, A. J., and F. H. Dodd. 1984. Reviews of the progress ofdairy science: mastitis control-progress and prospects. J. DairyRes. 51:481–512.

Bramley, A. J., and R. Foster. 1990. Effects of lysostaphin on Staphylococcusaureus infections of the mouse mammary gland. Res.Vet. Sci. 49:120–121.

Brantley, D. M., F. E. Yull, R. S. Muraoka, D. J. Hicks, C. M. Cook,and L. D. Kerr. 2000. Dynamic expression and activity of NFkappaBduring post-natal mammary gland morphogenesis.Mech. Dev. 97:149–155.

Family. *J Mammary Gland Biol Neoplasia*, 7:327-345.

Rupp R, Hernandez A, Mallard BA .2007. Association of Bovine Leukocyte Antigen (BoLA) DRB3.2 with Immune Response, Mastitis, and Production and Type Traits in Canadian Holsteins. J. Dairy Sci.,90: 1029-1038.

Sharma, B.S., Leyva, I., Schenkel, F. and Karrow, N.A., 2006. Association of toll-like receptor 4 polymorphisms with somatic cell score and lactation persistency in Holstein bulls. J. Dairy. Sci. 89, 3626-3635.

Sheehy, P.A., . Riley L. G., Raadsma, H. W. *et al.*, 2009. A functional genomics approach to evaluate candidate genes located in a QTL interval for milk production traits on BTA6. Animal Genetics .40 (4):492–498.

□□□

